THE BUSINESS SIDE OF VETERINARY MEDICINE

THE BUSINESS SIDE OF VETERINARY MEDICINE

What Veterinary Schools Don't Teach You

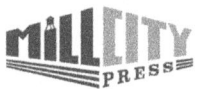

M. DUFFY JONES, DVM
TOM HARBIN, MD, MBA

Copyright © 2015 by M. Duffy Jones, DVM
& Tom Harbin, MD, MBA

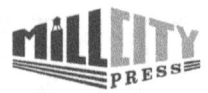

Mill City Press, Inc.
2301 Lucien Way #415
Maitland, FL 32751
407.339.4217
www.millcitypublishing.com

All rights reserved. No part of this publication may be reproduced, stored in a retrieval system, or transmitted, in any form or by any means, electronic, mechanical, photocopying, recording, or otherwise, without the prior written permission of the author.

ISBN-13: 978-1-63505-627-3

Printed in the United States of America

We dedicate this book to our families.
For Dr. Jones, to Courtney, Dawson, Grady, and Sydney for putting up with me on a daily basis.

For Dr. Harbin, to Ellen for putting up with me.

Contents

Introduction • 1

PART I: GETTING STARTED • 7
Chapter 1: Entering the Real World • 8
Chapter 2: Negotiating the Contract • 25
Chapter 3: Building a Practice • 35

PART II: LEARINING BUSINESS • 59
Chapter 4: Business Communication • 62
Chapter 5: Organizational Behavior • 72
Chapter 6: Marketing • 91
Chapter 7: Economics • 99
Chapter 8: Accounting • 103
Chapter 9: Business Law • 112
Chapter 10: Operations Management • 118
Chapter 11: Corporate Finance • 121
Chapter 12: Ethics • 133

PART III: YOUR CAREER • 137
Chapter 13: Issues in the Early Years • 138
Chapter 14: Are You Headed in the Right Direction? • 140
Chapter 15: Group Leadership • 150
Chapter 16: Transition to Retirement • 166

Introduction
By Tom Harbin
M. Duffy Jones

You're a veterinarian and you know a lot about medicine. But do you know about the real world? Did you learn anything practical in your training? Do you know how to plan for your life? If you're in training, do you know how to evaluate opportunities? If you're in practice, do you know how to manage, plan your finances, and think about the future? Have you chosen the right practice model for you and your family? Perhaps you're in academic medicine. Do you know how to lead a research team? Do you know how to get the most out of your practice?

Maybe you've been practicing awhile. Do you know how to increase your net worth? Can you chair a meeting and effectively lead your group? Are you planning for retirement?

Doctors learn a lot in vet school, but not enough. Only rarely will a course teach practical, useful, or pragmatic information to help with the myriad decisions that arise in day-to-day life. We wrote this book to fill the gap: to help doctors deal with the business aspects of veterinary medicine, to help doctors in training learn how to evaluate opportunities for the future, and to assist practicing doctors in dealing with the questions arising day-to-day and when planning for the future.

This book is adapted from a book written earlier by one of this book's coauthors, Tom Harbin, M.D., M.B.A. (henceforth, TSH), *The Business Side of Medicine: What Medical Schools Don't Teach You.* Dr. Harbin wrote his book after years of frustration with the lack of business training in medicine and after he completed an MBA at Georgia State University. Almost every professional school neglects to teach this information, not just medical schools, and much of the content of the book applies to other fields. Dr. Duffy Jones has practiced veterinary medicine for fifteen years and experienced the same frustrations. He has applied his hard-won experience as he adapted the book for his profession. Henceforth, if the pronoun *I* is used, it refers to Dr. Jones, and if *we* is used, then both authors are weighing in.

How to Use This Book

This book is important for doctors at all stages of their careers, whether in training or in practice. Part I deals with getting started after training: entering the real world, good citizenship in the new setting, and building a practice. Part II applies lessons learned from the different courses of an MBA curriculum to the issues that arise in a medical practice. Here we cover business communication, organizational behavior, marketing, economics, accounting, business law, operations management, corporate finance, strategy, and ethics. Part III covers the span of a medical career and the questions and decisions that arise in early, mid, and late career.

Why This Book?

You may have picked up this book for a variety of reasons. Perhaps you've thought the following:

"I went into medicine to be a doctor, not to do business."

"I didn't go to veterinary school to be in business; I want to take care of animals."

"I'm not interested in money; I just want to do research."

"All I want to do is treat animals. Let somebody else take care of the rest."

A 1987 *Wall Street Journal* article had quotes like these from a number of doctors.[1] The business aspects of medicine frustrated them and, along with managed care, defeated them. They left medicine unhappy, bitter, and with unfulfilled potential and wasted years of education. They were angry at the "system." But was their anger aimed at the right target?

More recently, an essay in the *New York Times* bemoaned the fact that the author now has to think so much about the financial aspects of medicine.[2] "We were trained to think like caregivers, not business people. The constant intrusion of the marketplace is creating serious and deepening anxiety in the profession."

Where did these doctors get the idea that they would be exempt from the forces that rule everyone else's lives?

---

1   Sonja Steptoe, "Dispirited Doctors," *Wall Street Journal*, 10 Apr. 1987: 19–21.

2   Sandeep Jauhar, MD, "A Doctor by Choice, a Businessman by Necessity," *New York Times*, 7 July 2009: D5.

What if they had been told since day one of veterinary school that they would need to know more than anatomy, pathology, and biochemistry, and that medicine is a profession that has business aspects that need to be learned? What if they had been educated about organizational behavior, finance, marketing, and business communication as well as the traditional subjects? What if their professional education had not only shaped their expectations about business realities, but also provided training about how to handle them?

You know the answer. Such education would have been wonderful and prevented much floundering and poor decisions, but we didn't get it; hence we wrote this book.

If you're completing your training, you may realize you have no idea how to evaluate a practice opportunity, look at an employment contract, judge a community, or choose a hospital. You also may not know your financial potential or how to finance your professional life.

Perhaps you're already practicing and you realize you have to do some things you never thought about: hire, fire, organize your patient flow, attract referrals, make patients happy with more than your medical skills, establish relationships with referring doctors, keep OSHA at bay, supervise fee collection, and decide which insurance company contract to sign.

Or maybe you've decided, as an increasing number of young veterinarians have, that you want to work for a corporate entity. You will still need to organize your professional activities, attract patients, satisfy referring veterinarians, write letters, choose and manage personnel, invest in a retirement plan, and negotiate within a corporate environment.

Some want an academic career. If so, you will need all the skills listed in the previous paragraph and more: building a team in the lab, handling the pressures of teaching, doing research and publishing while earning your salary from your practice, managing and motivating the employees in your area, etc. Young academic vets face some of the greatest challenges in beginning a career in medicine.

After practicing for about fifteen years, Tom Harbin entered the Executive MBA (EMBA) program at Georgia State University. For those two years he marveled at how relevant the various business courses were to his practice life and wished he had known about the material long before then.

Our central thesis in this book is this: there is a business side of veterinary medicine, and indeed all professions, the knowledge of which makes one a better doctor or academic. When you begin a practice or build a research program, you become the CEO of a small business. The CEO knowledge that you never were taught makes for better productivity, better patient flow and satisfaction, happier staff and family, and a more stress-free doctor. It makes for better team building, whether a practice team, an academic lab, or an entire academic department. It makes for better communication skills, written and verbal, for efficient meetings, and for ethical conduct. This material is just as important as medical knowledge and should be taught at some point during professional training. It currently is not, in part because school leaders themselves have no clue, and businessmen on the boards of universities don't make it happen.

In the *New York Times* article already referenced, the author states, "Something fundamental is lost when doctors start thinking of medicine as a business." We submit that medicine and business are not either-or propositions, that you can be a professional and take excellent care of your patients *and* still know how to handle the business aspects. Indeed, the more you master the business principles that apply in medicine, the better care you can take of your patients and the happier doctor you will be.

We will not be able to reproduce a two-year MBA curriculum in one book; moreover, each of us has experiences in our community that contribute to the knowledge imparted herein. For example, I began my practice as a one-doctor practice and over time grew that practice into a five-doctor practice. My real-world experience from start-up to large practice is critical for this book.

This book distills all those experiences into a reference manual for a lifetime in medicine, from beginning to end. We will go for the big picture—the principles, the vision, and how to think about issues. In addition, we will provide you with strategies for implementing your vision. We will not discuss tactics or the details of carrying out each strategy—you will find these details elsewhere, and they vary from state to state. We will teach you the questions to ask and the big issues to settle. We want you to avoid some of the frustrations both of us encountered, make better decisions, and learn the business issues of medical life. Ultimately, we want you to be better in your practice or academic life, less stressed, and more efficient. Your patients and staff will appreciate it, and you and your family will be happier.

PART I: GETTING STARTED

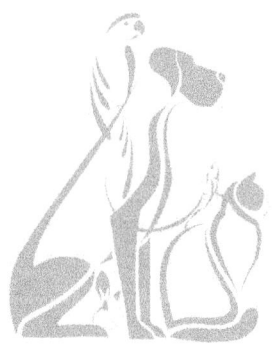

Chapter 1: Entering the Real World

It's the fall of your last year of training and you need to figure out the rest of your life. Thirty years ago, the majority of veterinarians entered private practice as solo practitioners. Now, the landscape has changed and the rate of change is accelerating. There are corporate options available that were not available years ago. Larger private practices allow one to become either a partner or just an associate. Internships and residencies offer advanced training. And finally there is still the solo practitioner. We will discuss the process of finding a private practice in detail, but these principles apply to those seeking an academic position or corporate employment.

Take the Long View

Before sending out résumés and talking to practices, spend time thinking about what you really want. We don't mean what salary you want in the first year of practice, even if that's first on your mind at the moment. Nor do we mean the details of where your office will be located and where the patients will come from. Where do you want to be ten years from now? What type of practice do you want for yourself: group, partnership, solo, associate, or corporate? Are you working full time or part time? Will you be the primary wage earner or a secondary wage earner? What geographical area will make you and your family happy?

You should always think about the long-term implications of a current decision. Decisions based only on short-term thinking can harm your long-term success. For example, you have two choices for a job. The first offers a generous salary the first year, allowing you a better lifestyle immediately, as well as the opportunity to easily pay down some of your debt. The doctor who founded the practice still owns it, and all the other doctors are well-paid associates. Several doctors have left the practice, but that's fine—you like everyone you have met and you're confident you can get along. A partnership of tight-fisted doctors runs the second practice. They don't offer a great salary the first year and they don't guarantee anything after three years. However, you will have the option to buy into the practice after those three years.

With just these facts in mind, which is the better choice? Of course it depends, but if you are going to be the primary wage earner, the second choice is better when you take the ten-year perspective. After ten years in the first job, you will have no ownership and you will still be an employee, with no effective voice in how your practice is run. The other doctors who left likely did so because they were unhappy. They wanted a say in the decisions that affected their daily lives and wanted to have ownership in an enterprise they added value to every day. Yes, you would make more money in the first few years, but your long-term earning potential is stunted. If you become unhappy and leave, the expenses—financially, emotionally, and otherwise—will far outweigh the higher initial salary. At the end of ten years in the second job, you're an owner and your partnership has probably brought in new doctors who have compensated you for the effort you made in building the practice. You have a say in the running of the practice and can help correct the inefficiencies and irritations that arise each year. You've maximized the earnings potential for your practice lifetime and have something you can sell when you decide to retire. You didn't make as much money as you wanted in the first few years, but now you're in much better shape.

Think about the long-term implications of any decision you make. Don't sacrifice the long term for imagined advantages in the short term. Make your career decision based on where you want to be in ten years, not two years. The next section discusses what factors to consider when contemplating your future.

Where?

Where do you want to spend the rest of your life? Close to where you trained or close to where you grew up? Big city, small town, or in the country? Where do you want to be ten years from now? Just as important, or possibly more so, where does your spouse want or need to be? Your spouse's job or your own specialty may dictate the choice. If you're a specialist, you will have to go where the specialty facilities and job openings are. Your choices are much more limited than general practitioners, who can go wherever they choose. You presumably accepted these limitations before you began your training, and you're stuck with them now.

When I was in school, the administration brought in working veterinarians in all fields to talk to us about the real world. These lectures constituted all the practice advice I ever received in a formal manner, and it was helpful. One of the pieces of advice was to live where your spouse / significant other will be happy. You are not the only one affected by the location of your practice. Your spouse has thoughts and feelings on this issue. If you do not consult your spouse in this decision, you may spend several years building your practice only to leave because your family would be happier elsewhere. You will have wasted several years and suffered the emotional price of moving to a new location and starting over. It would be far better to have anticipated where you and your family would be happy at the very beginning.

Before you spend time looking at a practice or academic opportunity in the area of your initial interest, ask about the potential for success in that area. In many popular areas of the country, notably California, Florida, New York, and other attractive urban areas, there are many veterinarians and vigorous competition. The atmosphere is cutthroat and aggressive. Is that you? Do you want to be in an area where you have to market, advertise, and truly hustle for patients? Does this fit your personality and approach to life? If it doesn't, you may discover after several years that you found the right place but cannot make a go of it financially. This is yet another consideration on the "where" of your search.

What?

Do you know what type of practice you want? Nothing is perfect; each type has advantages and disadvantages. Bear in mind that if living in a certain area takes the highest priority, you may have fewer choices in the type of practice you would like.

Solo Practice

I know that few will come right out of school and start a practice; however, if this is your ultimate goal, now is the time to begin thinking about this option. Do you want to be the only player in the enterprise or the exclusive decision maker? Do you hate meetings? Are you comfortable practicing without colleagues close at hand, handling the difficult problems by yourself? Do you have any business experience or at least some feel for running an office? If so, solo practice deserves consideration. In such a practice, you can locate your office where you want. You also set the efficiency level—that is, the number of staff helping you. Some doctors want helpers surrounding them. Some want to delegate tasks to nurses or assistants, where others want to do it all. The more helpers, the bigger the payroll and the greater the overhead, but the greater the volume of patients one can see. If you're solo, it's your choice.

You should consider the expense of being a solo practitioner. Start-up costs are higher because you need an office and have lots of equipment to purchase. The purchase of equipment will also be dictated by how you want to practice. If you are in a place where you see lots of emergencies, then you will need more in-house equipment, such as blood machines. If you are in a place where the outside lab can give you fewer than twenty-four hours' turnaround time on your blood work, then you might not need as much in-house equipment. Do you utilize ultrasound? If so, that is a big purchase. If you do not, do you have someone who does traveling ultrasound or a place close by, to which you can refer? Do you want to focus more on routine care or on treating medical or surgical cases? All of these factors will affect everything from the equipment you purchase to your hours of operation and the physical setup of your building.

Other considerations include the need to have coverage for weekend call. As a solo practitioner, will you take call or refer to an emergency clinic? What will your hours be? Will you have extended hours because you live in a community that is heavily commuter-based, or can you have more normal hours? Is your goal to start out as a solo practitioner, then take on an associate? Again, there are great joys of being a solo practitioner, but you have to love making tough decisions.

Associate

Do you want to settle into practice right away without having to hire a staff? Do you want a ready-made base of patients and others to share weekend duty? An associate position might be for you. Being an associate has many advantages, including having older, more experienced doctors around to help you learn the business side of veterinary medicine. These mentors will help you with medical cases as well and can be a great resource as you enter the real world. Being an associate allows you to focus on being the best veterinarian possible without any management headaches. Is working part time something that you desire? If so, being an associate may be perfect. However, there are disadvantages. You will not have much say in management decisions. Typically, the owner or management team sets office or hospital policy, so if you want to make changes, it might be difficult and involve convincing others of your ideas. Purchasing new equipment may be a challenge as well. You may not get the equipment that you need or want because the owner has other ideas for the hospital. Being an associate might be great for a short time as you learn how the real world of veterinary medicine works, but it may not be your long-term goal.

Owner

Do you want to own something and make decisions like a solo practitioner but want to have other veterinarians around? Maybe owning a larger multi-doctor practice is something you want. It can give you the ability to make the decision, but you will have the trade-off of trying to manage multiple associates and lots of staff. It can be the most financially rewarding, but you will spend more time being a manager than an actual veterinarian. If ownership is for you, then you have to decide how to get there. Do you start your own practice and hire your own associates as you grow, or do you look to buy into an existing practice? Each has advantages and disadvantages.

Corporate Employment

Do you want to share a practice and spend less than full time seeing patients? Do you want an eight-hour day of work and then to go home? Perhaps a corporate practice will suit you. In this setting, you have even less control over schedule setting and staffing and you build up no equity in your practice. You have no ability to sell your practice when you retire.

But you can move to another area more easily and you may enjoy benefits not offered in private practice. Your salary continues, at least short term, no matter your productivity.

As you can see, no practice opportunity is perfect. Each has advantages and disadvantages. Your job is to project yourself ten to fifteen years down the road, figure out what you want, and select the type of practice that suits you for the long term. If you truly don't know, realize that no decision is permanent and you can change your type of practice. It just costs you when you do.

Who?

If you've decided on solo practice, keep reading because you might need to be an associate for a few years before starting out on your own. If you want to be an associate and you know the general location where you want to be, you're now down to finding the practice that's best for you. Understand that outside of selecting a spouse, choosing a practice is the biggest decision that you will make for your adult life. You will spend as much or more time with these veterinarians as your family, and your happiness at home will depend on how you spend your workday hours.

Moreover, the community will judge you as much, if not more, by the practice as your own qualifications. You should find out as much about a prospective practice as you can by asking other doctors, both those in practice and those in academia. You should meet every member of the practice on at least two occasions. Once you are serious about a practice, your spouse should meet as many members and their spouses as possible. You should respect and ideally like the doctors in the practice. You will spend many hours with these people, and they will expect you to fit into the construct of the group, not the other way around. If you see something you don't like, don't think that you can go in as a new member and change the rules to suit your own needs. You will be expected to fit in.

How does the community at large regard your prospective practice? What is its reputation in the veterinary community? This key factor may be difficult for you to discover, but it's important. You will have to ask a number of doctors and listen carefully. In these litigious times, people are reluctant to speak frankly, especially to say negative things. You should ask members of the prospective practice what they consider their reputation to be. If you hear, "They [other doctors] don't like us, but we're good," or words to that effect, look into it and consider it a warning. Some practices have reputations for doing great medicine, where others do the minimum. Such group behavior becomes known in the veterinary community, and all members of the practice are looked at in a similar light.

If you're lucky enough to be considering several options in your desired area, one factor for the long term is the practice's efficiency and overhead. See the discussion under *Negotiating the Contract* in chapter two. A well-run group with lower overhead, all other factors being roughly equal, will provide greater financial rewards over the years should you be able to buy in. A corollary to this is the overall financial stability of the practice. A glance around the office can reveal glaring problems such as dilapidated furniture or out-of-date equipment, but it will take some direct questioning to uncover other details. If you have the potential to buy into the practice, ask even more questions. Ask if any emergency loans have been necessary or if there have been salary cuts to office personnel. You may meet the practice's banker along the way, especially if you will need a loan yourself. Talk to the banker about this issue. Most veterinary practices are stable, but when a recession hits, people reduce their discretionary spending. And to a degree, paying for veterinary care represents such spending. Some people will find a way to get rid of their pets or reduce paying for good care. When this happens, cash flow and loan repayments can suffer.

You may be hesitant to ask probing questions, but you should ask them anyway, especially if a future buy-in is an option. The group looking at you will or should ask similar questions about you, and you have every right to know everything about these practice details. Ask if any doctors have left in the past few years and why. Then go talk to the doctors that left and get their side of the story. Compare the answers. Check out the group with your faculty and at the hospitals in town. Ask, ask, ask. You cannot do enough of this type of due diligence. It's vital to your search.

If your research turns up red flags, pay attention. As we stated earlier, you will likely not hear out-and-out criticism as you talk to other doctors, and disparaging remarks will be understated. Don't let your desire to find a job blind you to problems. Make sure you listen carefully and chase down every negative remark. If you hear enough or you have a bad gut feeling, look elsewhere. It's far better to avoid a mistake than to land a job quickly.

Joining a Solo Practice

What if the practice is a solo doctor? First, find out if adding you to the practice is the first time for this practice. If there is a history of new doctors joining and then leaving, look out. This doctor is likely looking for cheap help and has no intention of keeping you on. Talk to each and every person who has left the practice. Talk to the staff if you can get a private moment. Scrutinize the employment contract for your rights. Be very careful before you commit.

If indeed your potential position is the first for the practice, you need to know if this constitutes a retirement move for the founding doctor or a way of growing the practice. If it's a retirement move, you should have a set way of buying in and a definite date on which you take over the practice. A non-compete for the retiring doctor should be part of the final contract. If you're buying the practice for a set price, you should own the practice and run the show at the end of the buy-in. If the retiring doctor changes his or her mind about retiring, the way in which that doctor stays, or indeed if it is allowed, should be up to you.

You should anticipate the opposite, i.e., the retiring doctor leaving before transitioning the practice to you. You will retain more patients if there is a long transition—a year optimally, six months at a minimum. The amount of time off during the transition period for the retiring doctor should be agreed upon, with price reductions for you if the conditions are not met. If the doctor leaves early, your investment is worth less, so you should pay less.

What if the doctor is young, busy, and wants to grow? Are you being hired as an associate or a future partner? If you're slated to be a partner, you should not expect to run the show, and the buy-in should be different from the scenario mentioned previously. The future of your earnings is less definite, at least as compared to eventually taking over a known income stream. Your buy-in should reflect this uncertainty and have provisions for reduction if the practice growth does not occur.

In this scenario, should you share power equally? Equal power sharing sounds democratic and fair, but problems can quickly arise. Someone needs to run the show. Employees quickly discover they can play one against the other if power is shared equally. Rarely do two people agree most of the time. So no, you should not expect an equal say in matters, at least not for a while.

The founding doctor should act as the CEO and should govern most of the important affairs and the daily office operations. After a relatively short time, you should expect to vote on big items such as adding new doctors, a large capital expense, or selling/merging the practice. You should read the next section even if you're joining a solo practice. Many of the principles apply to your situation.

Joining a Group Practice

How do you find out about practices in your desired area? If you want to stay in the area in which you trained or return to your hometown, you probably already know who the practices are, and you just need to find out which doctor is in charge of talking to prospective new hires. In these situations, one of your current professors can make some inquiries for you or tell you details you need to know. Make use of these resources. The final task of a training program is to assist you in landing the best possible job, so take advantage of this resource.

If you want to go to a totally new area and your teachers can't help you, it will take a lot of work to find the right practice. You can start by talking to the state's veterinary society. They can give you veterinarians in the area to talk with. They can typically guide you to good practices and good veterinarians with whom you can consult.

A good place to start your search is the AVMA (American Veterinary Medical Association) and the local veterinary medical association. Other good sources include the local referral or emergency hospital. They are in touch with local hospitals and usually know who is hiring. Consider doing relief work at the local emergency clinic. This will give you a view of the local landscape as well as the type of medicine practiced by each practice.

Still another resource, and a great one, is the Student Doctor Network (SDN, www.studentdoctor.net). SDN is a web community of students and trainees in a variety of disciplines including veterinary medicine. It hosts a number of forums to discuss many of the issues contained in this book—those involving medical students, residents, fellows, and those early in practice. Many of its participants began their involvement in medical school and have continued their participation into the practice years.

Don't necessarily be deterred by the lack of a job listing in a given area. If you have decided on a specific city and don't see opportunities, knock on doors. Call a doctor in each practice in that city. In some instances, a practice may be just starting to search, and your proactive call will hasten the process. In other situations, if you make it clear that, for whatever reason, you will be coming to that community, a practice may want to make room for you to avoid having a competitor spring up near them. In fact, I hired one of my best doctors in just this manner. She called and requested an interview. I told her I was not hiring but she persisted in wanting to meet me. She was so impressive that I did hire her and she has turned out to be a great doctor and asset to our practice.

Before the interview, do your homework. Know as much as you can about the individual doctors as well as the scope of the practice. How much are you expected to refer? Do you have to refer to in-house specialists or to one certain specialty clinic?

During the interview, do you click with at least some of the doctors? Do they seem to like each other? Does the group socialize after work? Many practices do not, but if this one does, your spouse's feelings and impressions take on even more importance. Your spouse will likely pick up on some things that you miss, so don't ignore that source of input.

Group Culture

When Dr. Harbin began his MBA studies, the faculty assigned a very dry book on the culture of organizations and made everyone read it before classes began. The class groaned whenever the book was mentioned in the organizational behavior course. But there was good reason in taking up the study of culture, and both of us appreciate the importance of culture more every year. Group culture rules everything. As one doctor said later, "Culture trumps strategy every time." When I began my career, no one ever talked about culture. I had no idea that different practices could have different cultures. If I had known about culture, it would have helped me understand the practices I worked in before starting my own.

Culture refers to the unwritten rules by which a group operates, including "the way we do things": the expectations of staff about behavior; how patients, vendors, and employees are treated; and the ethics of the group and how strictly the rules are followed. Culture determines all of these and more. We think of culture as the same as the ethics of the practice.

If you learned very conservative indications for testing or operating and join a practice with much looser ones, over time you will more closely mimic the group you joined. It will happen insidiously and almost without your realizing it. If the practice's norms are aberrant, you will either leave or become like your group. If you stay, you will become aberrant. You will not change the members of that practice by your different behavior. On the other hand, if your practice is conservative and you are too loose, either you will change or they will ask you to leave. The group will not change. Remember even as much as you try, you will not change the culture unless you are the owner, and even that might be hard. When Dr. Jones was younger, he thought that he could change culture. It led to frustration on his part and on the part of the practice owner for whom he worked.

The April 2, 2007, issue of *American Medical News*[1] quoted a study performed by the Cejka Search group and the American Medical Group Association to determine why physicians left a group practice. The study revealed that 51 percent of the time, the most common reason was poor cultural fit with the practice. This confirms the importance of culture as you evaluate a practice.

If you connect with the practices's culture, you and they will be happier, and your adjustment will be easier. So how do you find out about a group's or even a solo practice's culture? Ask and observe. Spend time at the practice. Watch how the staff treats patients—in most instances, their treatment of patients mimics the doctors'. Talk to referring doctors (if you are looking at a referral practice) and hospital administrators; look and be aware of what you want to know. Can you see yourself fitting in? Would you want your family treated this way? Is this how you learned to behave or want to behave?

Listen carefully to the doctors and staff during your interviews. What do they demand of you? What are their goals for you? How do they refer to clients and colleagues in the community—respectfully, scornfully, lovingly, or calculatingly?

Be aware of the importance of culture. Ask the doctors to describe their culture, although many will have no idea what you're asking. Try to schedule some free time in the office just looking and listening, if that's practical. Observations on such occasions can help reveal culture and true

---

1 Myrle Croasdale, "Gender, Age Factors in Physician Retention, " *American Medical News*, 2 Apr. 2007.

personalities. Ask and look. You cannot do enough of this type of diligence.

When the interviews have concluded, you should know whether you like and respect the practice and its culture, and what your duties will be. You should be happy and comfortable with all these factors.

Chapter 2: Negotiating the Contract

Now comes the challenging part: negotiating your contract. It's important that you have one, whether you're joining a solo practitioner, multi-doctor practice, or corporate practice. The days of handshake deals are over, and a contract protects you far more than it does the practice. When I first got out of school, I was so happy that someone hired me that I did not think about a contract. The owner told me I would have to work a few more Saturdays than the other doctors. In my mind, a few more meant maybe three or four more. As it turned out, to him it meant every Saturday for the first year! Because I did not have anything in writing, I was stuck. For ease of discussion, when I use the word *practice* in this or other sections, I refer to sole practitioner, multi-doctor, and corporate practice.

Initially, your main duty is to keep your word and show up to work. If you change your mind about joining the practice, it has little significant recourse against you. If you found the practice with the help of a recruiter or consultant, accept help from him or her with the basic issues in the contract. If you found the practice on your own, you may feel more comfortable with the help of a consultant when negotiating a contract. In the end, you will need an attorney.

The following text box lists the general provisions of a professional contract—including your duties and the group's duties.

> **GROUP'S DUTY TO YOU:**
> - Compensation
> - Facilities/Staff
> - Insurance
>   - Spouse covered?
>   - Dental?
>   - Disability?
>   - Life?
> - Vacation
> - Illness/Salary coverage
> - Termination
> - Death Benefits
> - Noncompetition terms
>
> **YOUR DUTIES TO THE GROUP:**
> - Loyalty
> - Records
> - Promoting the practice

Attorney

The practice has many duties to you, and they should all be spelled out. We are not lawyers and will discuss only a few of the issues that need to be negotiated. Moreover, every state's laws differ in some ways. You must have your own attorney, but be careful whom you hire. There are "can-do" and "can't-do" attorneys, and you need one who will give practical advice and find a way to craft a contract in the way you and your practice decide. This is especially true if you're negotiating the points without the aid of a consultant. I am very fortunate in that my wife's father is my attorney. Some people say never mix business with family, but he has been a tremendous asset. His basic approach is to keep things simple. His contracts are short and to the point. Many times very long contracts are confusing to both parties, so even if you did not marry into a family with a lawyer, find a lawyer who can make clear and concise contracts; it will be easier for both parties in the end.

If you get the nit-picking type who finds fault with the most basic of contractual provisions and insists on changing the wording of almost everything, you've made a mistake. You will turn off your prospective group and spend a lot of money. You might even cause so much anger that the practice rescinds its offer. This happened once to me when the contract discussions were so difficult that I realized the doctor would be a poor fit and took back my offer.

Don't ask your attorney to do the basic negotiating. You and one other person, usually the owner of the practice or the practice manager, should agree on the terms. The consultant or lawyer's job is to advise you on whether the terms are reasonable and then, once you have jointly decided the terms with the practice, to render those provisions into proper legalese, or review the work of the practice's lawyer. If the attorneys negotiate, the expense escalates and the fighting starts—usually to your detriment.

Any practice that has existed for any period of time has done this before and has a set way of bringing new doctors on board. In this situation, there will already be a contract you can review and the process of first-year salaries, terms of buying in, vacation time, etc. that has already been settled with your predecessors. You should not expect a dramatic departure from this process, and indeed, you will cause resentment if you insist on terms that are better than the doctors preceding you have received. So your job is to understand the issues, be sure you can live with them, then review and craft the terms of variable issues with your attorney. If certain terms are truly exploitive, you're joining the wrong practice. Don't try to change those terms, as you wouldn't be able to anyway; just find another situation.

Buy-In

The normal buy-in opportunity in the veterinary world involves buying an entire practice. There are very few partnerships in veterinary hospitals like there are in the medical field. In the medical field, doctors are allowed to buy into the practice and then become partners with others. Veterinarians tend to hold practices as sole ownerships and then sell the entire practice when they are ready to retire. So if you are looking for a job with buy-in potential, it usually means looking for a job where the owner is looking to retire or sell the practice. If the practice is not already a joint partnership, most will not consider making it one. In most instances, the only time a practice will consider going from a sole ownership to a partnership would be to ensure an exit strategy. If you should find a practice that offers eventual ownership without having to purchase the entire practice, they will have a buy-in provision that allows/requires you to invest in the practice. Again, an ownership opportunity, even in the case of an exit strategy, does not normally occur within the first few years of practicing. Many owners will want to work with someone at least five years before offering him or her a buy-in opportunity. If you are truly interested in buying into a practice, then have the timing of your opportunity to buy in spelled out. Some owners might either intentionally or unintentionally forget to allow you to buy in.

If you find the rare practice that will let you buy in, is it fair for you to pay for that opportunity? From the point of view of the practice, it's absolutely fair. There are significant expenses associated with starting and maintaining a practice. There is also considerable risk with starting a practice that you will avoid by buying into an established practice. You essentially skirt all these expenses and risks, and benefit from the considerable work and time expended by your predecessors. You start with a built-in patient base and see patients from day one. You receive a salary before the practice is able to collect the fees you generate. There is value in all this, and it's fair to compensate those who made it happen. Moreover, once you buy in and have some ownership, you will benefit from this arrangement and will in turn be paid for your investment by the doctors who join after you, should you allow it.

What's a fair price? The issues vary from practice to practice, and you will need a practice consultant or accountant to help out. There are many ways to evaluate a practice, and the ways practices are evaluated change over time. However, it is always good to have someone who is working for you and only for you go over the numbers and the evaluation.

There is not an exact science to any evaluation, and they can be swayed in either direction depending on whom the evaluation is for. I was very lucky to have a great accountant who knows a lot about the business of veterinary medicine. He was able to pick apart many of the practice evaluations that I evaluated when I was looking to buy a practice before eventually deciding to start my own. He worked for me and only for me, so I trusted his opinions and advice. He was a tremendous asset when looking at buying into a practice.

...

What gives a practice its value? If you're buying a practice, from an investment standpoint, most of the value derives from the retention of patients whose fees fund the earnings. To a lesser degree, the value comes from any expensive equipment. If you buy a practice three months after a doctor has died, the practice has relatively less value. If you work side by side with a retiring doctor for six to twelve months, get to know many of the clients, and retain the staff (which also keeps patients), the value of the practice is higher.

If you're joining a practice without purchasing the practice from a retiring veterinarian, the value is related to your expected income after becoming fully busy, and your share of the existing equipment. This assumes that any real estate is handled separately from the practice buy-in.

How you buy in can mitigate some of the risks of a purchase. If you pay an up-front amount, you take all the risk of patient retention and you have to pay with after-tax dollars that you borrow from the bank. If you pay a percentage of income for a few years, the retiring doctor takes the risk that you turn off the patients and he gets less. Moreover, you are paying with pretax dollars, a better deal for you.

Obviously, there are many variables, and thus many negotiating points. If you are uncomfortable with negotiating, you would do well to hire a practice consultant to help you. If you are joining a big clinic, you probably have little negotiating room since most clinics have a set way of buying in. Here, a consultant has much less to offer.

Investing in Other Assets

Many veterinary practices own the real estate of the practice. If the practice equivocates on allowing you to invest in the real estate, you should insist on it. If the other owners own something to which overhead dollars are paid and you never get to participate, you will be funding their net worth with your overhead contribution—a situation that will cause resentment over the years. Funding multiple investments in the first few years seems daunting at first, and it is. But your predecessors managed it and so can you. You're investing in your future, and you can do it.

Overhead Allocation

We discuss this in much greater detail in chapter fifteen, but it could be a negotiating point in a few situations. If that's true for you, review that chapter now and consider getting a consultant to help if you're at all uneasy with this topic.

Termination

While you and the practice are courting each other, you don't think about the negatives, such as termination, but it happens. What happens if you realize you made a mistake and joined the wrong practice? You should be comfortable that you will be treated fairly if you decide to leave for a distant locale and will not compete with the practice. The longer you have been with the practice, the more important this is. The terms of your leaving under this scenario should be fair to both you and the practice.

What if you're fired by the practice? If you're fired without a specific cause, you should get a severance check for several months' salary plus your contributions to a retirement plan. Many veterinarians fear they will work for several years, develop a practice, and then be terminated just before they have bought into the practice. This fear is unjustified in most instances, but there are practices, usually led by one dominating veterinarian, in which this occurs.

In most instances, the effort and time involved with recruiting a new veterinarian means that a practice has every intention of retaining you and wants to go through the recruiting process as rarely as possible. Remember, this is a marriage for the practice as well as for you. Recruiting a new doctor takes time, trouble, and expense. It's not a casual exercise for a practice. The best result from the practice's perspective is to hire someone who works hard, fits in, and allows the current doctors to live their personal lives without constantly recruiting people. Moreover, the process of firing a doctor is painful for the practice as well as the doctor. Practices do not go down this path lightly or frequently.

But there are abusive doctors who, despite their words, have no intention of sharing power or the economic pie. If you are the victim despite your best efforts, your only protection is the wording of the termination provision in your contract. Be sure you can live with the consequences.

Future Sale of Your Practice

If you are considering ownership or find the rare practice to buy into, will you be able to sell your practice if you retire or become disabled? What if you die? These questions are not top of mind when you are considering a practice but should be considered. All other variables being equal, if you can sell your practice at the end of your career, you are better off than if you just take your retirement plan and leave. If you buy a solo practice, obviously you can sell. If you join a big clinic, you most likely cannot, but you should get your accounts receivable or some consideration in addition to your retirement plan. What happens at the end of your career and what you can do with your part of the practice should be discussed now so that you know exactly all the agreements and expectations up front.

Noncompetition Agreement

The young doctor says, "You mean I'm supposed to sign away my rights to practice in my chosen area if things don't work out? The practice can just kick me out after I've worked hard for them for years? No way."

The established practice says, "You mean this kid wants to come in here, get to know all our clients and patients, and then be free to go across the street and compete with us? No way."

Non-competes can be tough. Some states prohibit them, so you can go to the next section if you're in such a state. Ethicists fuss over the issue.

From the point of view of a practice that wants to protect the enterprise it has built over time, a non-compete is essential. In my practice, you either sign one or we find someone else. End of story. I suspect this is true of most practices and support the idea of non-competes wholeheartedly. Here, a good attorney is essential. Courts have ruled that a non-compete must be reasonable in the area protected and the time that one has to obey the terms. The area covered has to be commensurate with the locale. Five miles may be fine in a highly urbanized area, but not enough in a small town. More than two years is unreasonable. In addition, you might want a monetary clause (liquidated damages) that allows you pay if you want to stay in the area.

If, as I previously discussed under *Termination*, most practices don't intend to kick you out, why have the non-compete? Not every doctor works out for a practice, for a variety of reasons. Some doctors have a poor work ethic, while some are disruptive and abusive to the staff. Some do not work ethically and choose to operate and bill excessively. Some are incompetent—even those from the best training institutions. There simply is no way to predict how a doctor will work out without several years of a relationship. No amount of wonderful letters of recommendation, board scores, grades in veterinary school, or training in the best of programs can predict how an individual will work out in practice. These will predict success the majority of the time, but not always, so the practice has to protect itself against making a mistake. If you like the practice and they like you, if you have seen no obvious problems, then sign the non-compete. It's the only way the practice will take you. Most of the time, you will toss the contract and the non-compete into a drawer and never look at them again.

Chapter 3: Building a Practice

Good Citizenship

You're in. Now what? If you joined a multi-doctor practice, how do you make sure you never have to look at that non-compete again? What can you do to make sure that your practice wants to keep you around? We tell young doctors that we will judge them on two fronts: how they practice medicine and "group citizenship."

This chapter discusses citizenship. The principles apply to every type of practice: solo, multi-doctor, corporate, or academic. The vision that should guide you is to be a good citizen of your practice, and always to be ethical, productive, and cooperative.

Practicing medicine is or should be the easy part. After all, that's what you have been learning for the past eons. You have learned the *what*, for sure. What to do when you're confronted with a disease or a problem has been the focus of all your training. Hopefully you have also learned the *when*: when to test or operate and, just as important, when not to. Knowing the *when* means having judgment, and you will gain more of this as you begin to practice and make mistakes, as we all do. We respect conservatism and ethics. If a young doctor operates on every vomiting dog, he or she will not last in my practice. If excessive and unnecessary testing and surgery indicate that a young doctor is more interested in income than the patients' welfare, the doctor will soon be gone. Ethical and conservative groups, at least ours, will tolerate a wide variety of personalities, as long as the proper treatment of patients occurs.

Your practice will assume that you can practice quality medicine. They will find out how willing you are to work hard. Are you happy to see patients late in the day? Are you willing to hustle? Are you willing to talk to owners in the lobby and on the phone? Are you willing to show up even when the schedule is light, to see the emergency work-ins even if it's lunchtime?

So you're a good doctor in all aspects, but what about this group citizenship stuff? Practices need cooperative, pleasant colleagues—not poisonous individuals who sow discord. In a practice, you can't have your way all the time, and you have to give up some of your desires for the good of the organization. Likewise, when the practice votes on something, you follow it—even if you voted against it. You may need to do some chores yourself to keep the overhead low. And nobody likes people who feel compelled to comment on every issue in a meeting so they can hear themselves talk.

You get the picture. Some people are just not cut out for group practice and don't realize it until they get into such a situation. These people vote one way at a practice meeting and go another way the following day. They scurry about, complaining about the most minor of issues, and throw poison into every meeting. Who needs it? Certainly not a happy practice that wants to take care of patients during the day and devote the least amount of free time to meetings and conducting the business affairs of the enterprise.

In sum, you owe your new practice the proper quality of medicine and good citizenship, civility, and good manners. You do your part, and you will stay forever.

Attracting Patients

You're a good doctor and a good citizen. You've arrived at the office, ready to go, ready to be a rookie for the last time in your life. Now what? How do you fill that schedule?

If you're solo, you have a mountain to climb. If you're joining a multi-doctor practice, you probably have a few patients to see, but likely not a full slate for the day. Most doctors have a period of months in which they come to the office but are not fully busy seeing patients. Now is the time to build the practice, as well as to establish good habits and organizational skills.

One cliché of attracting patients revolves around the three *As: Availability, Affability, and Ability*. If you're in a practice, the doctors assume you have the ability or they would not have hired you. The other two *As* are for you to learn.

Availability

You're the one with holes in your schedule, so let the front desk and other doctors know you want to see work-ins and emergencies. They will be glad not to burden their busy schedules with extra patients. Some of the biggest fights in our practice (at least when we don't have young doctors starting out) have concerned allocating the emergency patients who need to be squeezed in during busy days. The other busy doctors are happy to be relieved of the perceived burden of seeing extra patients.

You should make a point of letting all the doctors and staff know that you are dedicated to building your practice and you want to see the patients they don't want to see. Don't assume they know it. In fact, don't assume they're even aware of the exact date of your arrival. Months pass between the days of your interviews, your decision to join the practice, and your first day of work. The bigger the practice, the less aware many members are of your beginning date. They know generally that you will come when your training ends, but they don't know when you have it worked out. You should schedule some personal time with doctors after your arrival so you can tell them personally of your willingness to hustle.

While you are meeting with each of the doctors, pick a mentor. If you're reading this book, you realize the deficiencies in your education. Having a mentor you can trust and who can guide you in the politics of the group, hospital, or community will be invaluable. Model yourself and your practice after that doctor. Ask questions, even if they seem simple. Watch them to learn how to communicate. Make sure to watch how patients and employees are treated. Learn as much as you can.

Don't stop with the doctors, since they rarely control the day-to-day flow of patients. Let the staff member who takes the phone calls and has to allocate the patients know your desires. You will make that person's life a lot easier, at least until you get so busy that you can't take on all the emergencies. Learn who the key employees are, and if they like and respect you, they will give you referrals. The doctors and employees will be watching you in these first few weeks and months, and the impressions you give them will last.

As busy as you may think you are in the first few months of practice with moving and settling in, seeing patients for the first time, etc., you will never be less busy. You will never have more free time than during these months. Make sure the practice sends out an announcement that you have arrived. A little local PR can go a long way in getting you new clients.

Attend as many local and civic events as possible. Get to know everyone in your neighborhood and those you meet at other social gatherings. If you have children in a preschool or grade school, make sure the other parents know what you do. People like to do business with people they know, so the more you are known in the community, the faster your practice will grow.

After you have done all this, make sure you are truly available. Don't let your support staff undermine you. If it's 11:30 a.m. and your tech or nurse wants to go to lunch on time, that person will say no when the question of your working in a patient comes to them. Insist on seeing that patient. Emphasize to your tech that filling your schedule with work-ins takes precedence over on-time lunch. Be sure the employee who takes the initial phone calls and has the duty of persuading someone to see these patients knows you want to see them. Check periodically to be sure there is no subversion of your wishes. Listen with a third ear to the phone conversations of your techs, and if you hear, "Oh, send that person to lunch. We will see them this afternoon," or some such delaying comment, insist on seeing the patient then. The same goes for late afternoon or the inevitable phone call on Friday afternoon. Make sure your front desk gets the phone calls to you. Without your knowledge, staff will erect barriers that constrict your availability. Don't let that happen.

Affability

It has been said for years, and the Mayo Clinic recently confirmed it: patients judge you by your bedside manner, not your professional ability.[1] Having no way to judge the technical aspects of your care, they judge by how you treat them.

When you walk in the room, introduce yourself if this is the first time with that patient. Shake hands with every person in the room, and greet them. Make a little small talk before you get down to business. Sit forward, at eye level with the pet's owner, and listen while you go over the history. Interact with the patient. Sometimes the dog or cat is friendly and wants to interact, and some others want to hide. If the pet wants to interact, you can be petting the dog while talking to the owner; if the pet wants to hide under the chair, then take a good history before you examine the animal.

You will, of course, deliver the best technical medical care you can to that patient, but owners want more. They don't want a brisk, take-it-or-leave-it message; they want full explanations and answers for all their questions, spoken in a caring manner. If you promise to call them later, make a note

---

1 Bendapudi, et al., "Patients Perspectives on Ideal Physician Behaviors," *Mayo Clin Proc* 2006;81(3):338–344.

in the chart and do so. If they mention a vacation before the next visit, make a note and ask them about it on that next visit. They will be impressed with your memory, and only a tiny minority will figure out that you made that chart note. Within the bounds of reality, give reassurance.

Know the unasked questions present in every visit and, if appropriate, give reassurance on that issue as well. Realize and anticipate the issues that don't arise. When you address them prospectively, you will have a grateful owner.

When you are with the owner, give plenty of time for questions. The issue burning in the owner's mind is usually the third or fourth concern they mention or ask about. If you focus on the first question and ignore the third, you will not give satisfaction. Learn the formal steps of reassurance therapy.

Give perspective to the owner. I hear questions and issues about which I have no idea but that I can put into a category. For example, if the owner has given a symptom for which there is no diagnosis, one answer is "I don't know." While this is honest, it's not always satisfying to a owner. Instead, answer in a manner that lets patients know you are looking out for them. "I don't know, but whatever it is, it's not serious" or, "I am not sure, but let me think if I can relate that specific concern to this current problem or investigate to see if we have another problem going on" would be more satisfying answers.

Be honest, especially when the condition is critical. If a patient is truly sick or dying, the owner is usually aware of it. If you sugarcoat the prognosis out of concern for the owner's feelings, you cheat that owner. If you acknowledge how truly serious a situation is and then figure a way to help the owner deal with it, you make a friend. If the owner is struggling with the decision about euthanasia, then tell them honestly what you would do if it were your own pet. Give them the reasons for that decision, but also listen. If they are not at the point of making that decision, make sure to offer them alternatives if possible. Often just the passage of time helps them with the decision.

One particular type of owner will challenge the dictum to spend enough time and answer all questions. This is the highly anxious but less intelligent person. They will tie you up for as long as you have, sucking all the energy out of you and totally wrecking your schedule. They will ask questions for hours and leave complaining that the doctor didn't spend enough time with them. They have no idea that you gave them far more time than the other 99 percent of your patients that week. Once you have identified such a patient, you can block off extra time or you can promise to call them after hours, explaining that you have to see other patients. In my experience, if you spend enough time in the first few encounters, such a person will calm down and take less of your time in the future.

Ability

Everyone assumes you have the ability. After all, this is what your veterinary training has given you to the exclusion of the topics covered in this book. Be aware that you have a lot of education but little to no experience. You may know the medical facts, but you haven't seen the full spectrum of diseases. You know how to do a test or procedure, but you may not know when and when not to do it. You don't have judgment yet, but you will, and you will gain it by making mistakes. By making these mistakes, you can learn from them, minimize them in the future, and learn how best to handle them. If you have partners, turn to them for help. They know what you are going through and don't expect you to have all the answers. They will respect you all the more when you ask for help in tough situations. If the inevitable bad outcome occurs, you will have someone to share the misery with, and it won't look like the rookie got in over his or her head.

In short, be conservative. Most patients and owners don't want surgery unless they really need it, and you will see palpable relief when you tell them that a given procedure can wait. The last thing you want is a poor outcome in someone where the original indications were iffy. This is bad not only for the patient, but for your reputation. Likewise, don't order every test in the book for every patient. Make sure you are running the appropriate tests for that patient. Not running a test when needed because you are worried the client does not want to pay for it can be as bad as running too many tests. Clients are looking to you for judgment and advice on the key tests, especially if they are invasive or expensive.

Communication Skills

This is one of the most important aspects of our field but is very often overlooked. Besides making good, sound medical judgments, you are expected to be able to communicate these judgments to a variety of personalities and listening styles. You will have to learn to adapt your presentation to the kind of person in front of you. Some owners want only the facts about their pet's condition and want clear choices on what to do. Others want to discuss more of the emotional side of the issue, and you will have to change approaches from fact-giver to listener and be more supportive. If you cannot explain to owners what is going on and why they need to perform these medical tests, you will be working against each other as a team to figure out the pets' medical problems. Watch as more seasoned doctors in the practice communicate with clients and see how they do it. It takes time and experience to deal with the many different types of personalities out there.

You will also have the joy of dealing with staff and their many personalities. You will have to develop your communication style and leadership style so that you can get the employees to do what you need them to do. Everyone has a style that works for them, but you do have to alter your style based on the personalities of staff members. If you are a matter-of-fact speaker who expects people to see things that need to be done and do them, working with a very sensitive personality is going to be hard for you. With sensitive people, not only do you need to communicate very clearly what you need done, but you also should give them praise when they accomplish that task. If you continue to work in your matter-of-fact manner, the sensitive employee will think that you do not like them and become stressed out. So remember, communication not only deals with clients but also with staff.

Organizational Skills

SEEING PATIENTS

You serve three masters as you go through your day: your schedule, your patients, and the clients. Naturally you want your schedule to go smoothly and your day to end on time. Your staff wants this more than you and will work to keep you on schedule. We have observed a good number of young doctors begin practice. The common complaint of staff is that they're too slow. They spend too much time with patients and the day drags on. Now, it's better to start off spending too much time with clients and patients and learning how to gracefully end the encounter than the opposite. After some months, the young doctor learns how to keep a schedule and make clients and patients happy. Be sure staff schedules appropriately as you learn this process.

Your clients and your patients, the second and third masters of the day, want you to see them on time and answer all their questions as if you had all day: two conflicting desires from the standpoint of your schedule. How do you learn how to reduce time with clients and patients yet make them feel satisfied with their visit? Learn how to use your staff. Have your nurse or tech take a lot of the history. Then you concentrate on the details key in the history that are pertinent to that visit. This also goes for instructions about medications: have your nurse go over them and send the patient out with written instructions. Studies have shown that most clients judge a visit by the total time taken with them, not just the doctor time. If someone spends time with them to be sure they understand their disease and treatment, and that person is caring, then within reason, that person does not have to be the doctor. You learn these efficient steps without sacrificing reassurance while satisfying clients and patients as discussed under *Affability*.

Organizing Your Life

You have a great filing system and can lay your hands on any item you want, quickly and easily. When you sit down at your desk, you have a list of things to do either at the phone or at the computer, so you can knock off a few items on your to-do list in those in-between moments. Likewise when you are out in the car doing errands, you have a to-do list for these occasions and can accomplish a number of pesky tasks on the same trip. You are totally organized, right?

Despite fervent wishes and multiple attempts, all of my tries at getting organized failed until I (TSH) was sixty years old and read David Allen's book, *Getting Things Done: The Art of Stress-Free Productivity*. He has a common-sense, logical approach to daily organization and makes the point that his system reduces stress by reducing clutter and clearing your mind of remembering the little things you have to do. By the time I adopted his system, my home office and work office were so disorganized that it took hours to de-clutter and get all the filing done. I wish I had discovered a system earlier. Allen's is not the only system out there, but it is the one that worked for me, and I recommend it. If you have another system, great; the point is to have a formal system that works for you. The earlier you get your files organized and you adopt a system for documenting all the things you need to do, the easier the job will be and the more years of reduced stress you will enjoy. Getting organized is another goal to accomplish in the early months of practice, before you get fully busy.

Good Habits

While you have time and inclination to make a good start, cultivate the habits discussed herein.

Conduct

You've come to a new community or have assumed a new status within your old community. You're a new professional, striving to establish a practice. How do you act? Do you take out ads in the paper? Drive a flashy new car or buy an expensive house? As good and exalted as your training may have been, it's all over. No one cares but you and your parents. You're a rookie all over again—hopefully for the last time, but nevertheless a rookie. In the eyes of the established members of your city, you're a newbie, likely one of many, struggling to establish yourself. They have seen a good many like you through the years, some failing, some succeeding. They'll be watching your behavior.

Do you drink too much at parties? Do you wear a white coat in the office? Like it or not, people will be scrutinizing your personal behavior and comparing it against their expectations. There are exceptions, but most clients want their veterinarian to wear a white coat and dress conservatively. Clients, fellow veterinarians, and neighbors don't want to see wealth flaunted or their new veterinarian intoxicated. They don't want wild variations of facial hair, tattoos, or pierced body parts. The more outlandish your dress, appearance, or behavior, the more egocentric clients will (accurately) judge you to be. Clients want veterinarians to be patient-centric, not egocentric.

So take an honest look in the mirror and compare what you see to your community. If you trained in California and now you're in Ohio, you might notice some differences, both in personal appearance and dress. You're in a new culture now, and the more you fit in, the happier your new clients will be.

Community Service

You've worked extremely hard during your training, and your debts prove it. Somebody owes you something, and now is the time to get it. These are feelings common to all of us who have gone through the hard years. Some express them in their behavior more than others. Actually, you have been subsidized to a significant degree, even if you paid your way. Who made up the gap between your tuition and the full cost of your education? Many times, the federal government, the state, your local community, or donors to your university—the citizens and foundations of your city—did. What do they want? Why did they pay these dollars? It's likely because they want good veterinary care for the community. They don't demand it, but they would also look favorably on your contributing time to various nonprofit agencies and training programs.

We believe we owe our community a degree of service. Even though we worked hard and achieved a lot by our own efforts, we were helped along by financial subsidies, and now we're granted high status in our community. If we give back by working with the agencies and do some teaching, we retain our status. If we collectively turn our backs on the community and focus only on our own incomes, we will lose that status over time. In many countries, veterinarians struggle with poor pay and low status. The current privileges granted to veterinarians by US society are not guaranteed to last forever.

In addition to feeling good about ourselves and contributing to the high regard afforded veterinarians, community service and teaching can help a practice grow. You will get to know community leaders who can direct clients your way. You won't regret your years of service, and you will never have more time for these activities than during your early years of practice.

Finances

You've been sacrificing for years, making less money than many of your college friends who goofed off while you were killing yourself in labs and difficult courses. You just signed a contract and your income will at least double or triple, if not more. You might think now is the time to buy all those things you've wanted: a new car, a big house, a boat, or whatever you want. You've sacrificed long enough.

Yes, you've sacrificed and you're almost there, but hold on—at least for a little while. Most young veterinarians have debts to pay, and those need to be factored in. Your taxes are going up, and you won't net as much income as you thought when you first looked at that contract. So you need to know how much extra net income you will have, and it won't be as much as you want. Do you have to buy some professional equipment or buy into the practice? What about a new wardrobe for the office? Do you have moving expenses? You will have extra expenses of some sort to go along with your new job and status in the community. Find out about these expenditures first, and then factor them into your new net income.

Establish the good habit of financial discipline now. The main feature of this discipline is controlling your spending. As tempted as you will be to spend all your disposable income, do not. Begin living below your means now and be careful about where the dollars go. First, as previously mentioned, get an idea of your new net income after your inevitably higher taxes and deductions, if applicable, for pension contributions. You may need the help of a professional, but here you have to be careful. They all want to sell you something. Along the way, they may give you good advice, but they are not attracted to you because of your personality and character. They're in the business of extracting fees for their services, and you're no exception. Whether it's a banker, an insurance agent, a financial planner, or whomever, they want you to do business with them so their income can go up. Be sure, to the best of your ability, that their primary interest is doing a good job for you and then getting a fee, just as your approach to serving patients should be.

How do you choose? Ask your other doctor coworkers and ask the practice owner. Talk to the practice accountant and banker and see whom you like. At this stage, you don't need investment advice, you need to learn how to forecast your income and manage your spending.

At the simplest level, there are three lines of dollars for you to consider. The top line represents your income, and you'll spend most of your time generating the top line. The second line is your spending, and you and your spouse should carefully monitor this line. The third line, the bottom line, is your net income. Your goal is to generate a bottom line, then learn what to do with it.

All of your training and most of this book's advice concerns your top line. We want you to generate a good top line, ethically and professionally, with your clients' and patients' welfare as your primary consideration. But at the end of the day, we want you to generate a bottom line, and limiting your spending achieves that ultimate goal. Spending does you in. As your income goes up, you begin to consider buying things that formerly were so out of your reach you didn't even think about them. You will always, no matter how much you earn, very easily be able to outspend your income. Don't do this. Know what you're doing and what effect it will have on your long-term plans.

Before you can spend those precious leftover dollars, you need to consider some specific issues: debt repayment, insurance, and retirement planning.

Debt Repayment

Many veterinarians end their training with considerable debt, and now it must be repaid. One question you may have is how quickly you must repay the debt. You probably have a loan with a set payback schedule and interest rate. You haven't lived it yet, but you will see business cycles in which interest rates for loans fluctuate considerably over the years. Your loan may have a great rate compared to what's currently available for you, or it may be very high. Here, the advice and help of your banker can help. If you now must begin paying back a loan with a high rate compared to what you can get currently, you may want to pay off the current loan completely by getting a new loan at lower rates and a monthly payment that's easier for you to handle. Whatever the case and your ability to refinance, these payments will have an impact on your bottom line.

Insurance

You will need both disability and life insurance. The odds of becoming disabled for a significant period of time are much higher than your dying, and you need the income protection—especially if you're the sole breadwinner for your family. Have you read your employment contract lately? If you have one, it should provide your monthly salary for a specified period of time, usually a few months, if you become disabled. These payments usually cease after three months, and here your disability insurance should kick in. If you are in solo practice, you can forecast how long you can stay afloat from your accounts receivable.

Disability Insurance

What should you do now? Get the best individual coverage that you can from a top-rated company. Get as much income coverage as you can from these types of policies, and then go for group insurance. Investigate group policies from the AVMA or your state medical association. Get good advice from a professional you trust. Have a few different people give you quotes to find out what is the best policy for you and your family.

Finally, if you pay your premium with after-tax dollars, the payments will be free of income tax. The payments are low enough already, so don't succumb to the temptation to pay for it through your practice with pretax dollars, as you will reduce the payout even more by income tax fees.

Life Insurance

The younger you are when you get life insurance, especially term, the cheaper it is. You owe your family a sustained and consistent lifestyle in the event you die. So get a lot of inexpensive life insurance and make sure your spouse and children can stay in your home and get a good education. Any number of insurance agents will approach you as you get established. Your problem will be finding a good excuse for saying no to those knocking on your door. You can't and shouldn't use them all. The easiest out is to use the agent who services your practice, after you make sure your colleagues are happy with that person and not contemplating a change.

How much? A big enough sum so that when it's invested in very conservative instruments, the income will allow your family to live in a nice home, receive an education, travel, and live the lifestyle you wanted to provide for them. It's more than you think. A million dollars yielding 6 percent a year provides $60,000, pretax. In mid-2015, no conservative financial instruments yield anything close to 6 percent, and the lower the yield, the more coverage you need. You will need several million dollars, depending on where you live, other sources of family income, state and federal tax rates, the need for private education or not, and other factors unique to you. Don't forget about inflation. A 3 percent inflation rate halves the value of the current dollar in twenty-four years and halves it again in another twenty-four. If you die at a young age, your spouse could easily live another fifty years. Do you want to relegate your loved ones eventually to live on 25 percent of current income? Obviously, the preceding is grossly simplified and should be refined by good advice aimed at your specific circumstances, but this should get you thinking.

Hopefully, you will never need either of these types of insurance coverage, and if you do, it may be many years down the road. We favor using only the best-rated and the longest-lived companies for your individual policies. It's false economy to go with the cheapest premium from a fly-by-night company that no one has heard of—it may fail right when your family needs help. Financial needs change as you proceed along, and you will need to periodically reexamine your coverage.

Retirement Planning

You won't believe we're saying this, but it's now time to prepare for your retirement. You will need to know the amount of the contributions to your pension plan. If you work for a corporation, this may be partially or fully paid by your company, but for most professional practices, these amounts are deducted from your gross salary. In most practices, you have no choice, but if you do have a choice, go for it, even when your take-home pay is reduced. If your practice agreement allows you to opt out for a few years, don't do it.

Why begin contributing for retirement? Why not spend money now, while you're young and healthy? Most people think that retirement will take care of itself, but no, it will not just magically happen. Most veterinarians have no one but themselves to pay for their retirement. Social Security will provide minimal help, and no other organization will pay you. One reason to begin your pension payments now is due to the discipline it involves. Now is the time to develop financial discipline, meaning preparing for your future years and not outspending your net income.

Second, a pension plan is the best tax shelter going. You don't pay tax on your contribution or the gains until you retire and take the money out to live on. This means a lot. If you get $100 in income, you will pay from $30 to $45 in taxes, depending on your bracket and state tax. If you put all of that $100 to work for you in a tax-deferred plan and you do it early, the return will astound you. Why? Through the magic of compounding.

Third, compounding works for you the earlier you start. If $100 appreciates at 6 percent, it will be worth $769 in thirty-five years. If you wait fifteen years to begin saving for retirement, your first $100 contribution will be worth only $321 in thirty-five years. The longer you allow compounding to work for you, the more you have for retirement. The last thing on your mind is finishing your career, but retiring will surely enter your mind when you have been practicing for thirty years or so. You may stop working when you are sixty, or you may never quit, but you want the choice when that time arrives.

> ### COMPOUNDING IN REAL LIFE
> - Assume $30,000 can be contributed each year starting at age thirty, with a 6 percent return.
> - If contributions begin at age thirty, $30,000 annually will grow to $2.7 million by age sixty.
> - If contributions begin at age forty, $30,000 annually will grow to $1.4 million by age sixty.
> - If you decide to delay the contribution, $30,000 will be worth $16,500 after tax, assuming 39 percent federal income tax and 6 percent state tax.
> - If you delay contributing until age forty, you have gained $165,000 in net income ($16,500 x 10), but given up roughly $1.3 million in retirement plan value at age sixty.

This is highly simplified and ignores inflation, but it shows the power of compounding over time.

Fourth, you are building a nest egg in case of disaster or disability. As discussed, some period of disability and the inability to earn a living is much more likely than early death. You should get as much disability insurance as you can, but you will find that it does not cover your income to an adequate degree, especially your future greater income. If you become disabled for a relatively short time, insurance plus savings and loans can keep you going. If you become disabled for life, you will be scrambling to maintain your lifestyle, and you will be grateful for any dollars in your pension plan, since you will be able to tap into this source without penalty.

So go out and get the necessary insurance coverage, net out your income after these outlays, your pension contributions, your higher taxes, and any other necessary and unavoidable expenses, and see what you have left. You will need to project this over several years since you can't begin contributing to your pension plan in the first year, in most situations. It won't be as much as you imagined or as much as you want, but it will keep you going to the office and hustling to get your practice off the ground.

And last, as soon as you can, begin a savings program outside your pension plan, putting aside dollars for emergencies, short-term disability, investments, and a down payment for a home. Then you can enjoy what's left over. You've earned it!

We've emphasized financial discipline and the need to establish these good habits, and now we can discuss the importance of having fun as you go along. Hopefully you will have a long and prosperous career followed by a happy retirement, but these are not guaranteed. Have some fun along the way, in case the way is shortened or damaged in some unpredictable fashion. Take some time off. Spend time with your family. Develop outside interests. You can do these while maintaining financial discipline and without building up crushing debt.

PART II: LEARNING BUSINESS

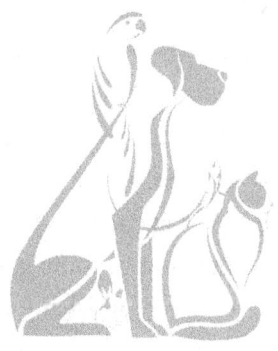

So you've been in practice for a while now and you have implemented the skills and processes that we have recommended. You're getting busier and busier, and the other veterinarians no longer consider you a rookie. Now they want help from you on the business side of the practice. You've been coming to the monthly meetings and you've sat through a year-end meeting or so but without full understanding of the issues or the reports you see. When you are asked to interview someone as a prospective employee or partner, you probably don't know which questions you are allowed to ask and which are forbidden.

Or perhaps you're on the board of a nonprofit agency and you get those financial reports every month. You may well not know what they mean or the difference between an income statement, a balance sheet, or a budget and how they relate to the mission of the agency.

You've sat through meetings—some good, some painful. One day you will be at the head of the table as the chair. Do you know the ins and outs of running a good meeting?

You're starting to get some money in your pension account. Do you know about investing, and the difference between a stock and a bond? Your neighbor wants you to invest in his business, and it looks like a winner. You would probably like to know how to tell how good it really is.

Your practice is thinking about a new satellite office and a new doctor. What's the long-term goal of the group? Have you ever had a formal strategic planning session? Where's the plan? Has anyone looked at it since it was printed and put in a drawer? You know when to write a memo or e-mail, when to make a phone call, and when to see someone face-to-face, and the different impact each type of communication makes on the recipient.

If you answered yes to any of the above, you've probably had some business training. If you answered no to the above, then you're in the majority, floundering your way through the issues that confront you weekly.

This is where help from someone with business training can be a tremendous asset.

The chapters of this part will summarize the pertinent points of the various courses in the MBA curriculum as they relate to a life in veterinary medicine. This material is not only for those just beginning practice but should apply to you throughout your practice life.

Chapter 4: Business Communication

You're talking to people all day long—patients, staff, employees, partners, and outsiders in the community. How you do it is important. It can make or break an exam and also make a difference to the client about wanting to come back. A great book about communication comes from Jerry Dibble: *Communication Skills and Strategies: Guidelines for Managers at Work.*

The most powerful way to communicate is face-to-face. Dibble calls this "full-channel communication." Several components contribute to the message received, and, surprisingly, the words you say comprise only a small part of the message—7 percent in fact. Your voice inflection delivers 28 percent of the message, and your body language, especially eye contact, sends the rest of the message. Thus, 65 percent of full-channel communication is nonverbal and depends on what you do when you're in front of someone.

> **Full-channel Communication:**
> 65% - Body language, eye contact
> 28% - Voice inflection
> 7% - Words

So look people in the eye. Put energy and expression into your voice. Don't spend your energy trying to find just the right words while you fidget with the chart or the meeting agenda. Words matter less than you think, and eye contact and emotion matter more. Make sure you're at eye level with the client, and lean forward while making eye contact. Your words are important but are forgotten quickly, and the emotional impact of your message will linger much longer.

A face-to-face meeting is full-channel but not possible for all the times you need to communicate something. You want to have such a meeting under the following circumstances:

1. The issues are sensitive.
2. There are several sides to be considered.
3. You need immediate feedback or you need to be sure others understand what you have to say.
4. You want maximum impact.

If a telephone message is appropriate or the only communication possible, remember that you lose 65 percent of a full-channel message, that related to body language and eye contact. Voice inflection becomes more important, so you need to project more energy and enthusiasm. You need to speak forcefully, perhaps more than in a personal meeting.

If you initiate the phone call, plan ahead of time. Know the points you want to get across and be organized. At the end, summarize the actions you will take and those you expect the listener to take.

Communicating with Clients

Here's one scenario: The doctor enters the exam room, looks at the chart, and addresses the client while standing and looking at the chart. The doctor does not look at the pet. The doctor tells the client the test results, medication instructions, and when to return. Then he's out of the room and on to the next one.

Here's another: The doctor enters the same room, looks the client in the eye while shaking hands, and then does the same for every family member in the room, including children. The doctor asks the child how old she is, makes small talk about the client's latest vacation, prompted by a chart note made on the previous visit. He examines the pet, even though the lab values make an exam moot. The doctor sits down, facing the client directly, and interacts with the client while explaining the diagnosis and the treatment. The staff writes down the treatment plan, as most people forget the details of what the doctor tells them.

You can easily imagine which scenario generates a positive reaction and which situation would score the highest on the client satisfaction survey received a few weeks later. When I began practice, I was much closer to scenario one. It took pointed remarks by a few clients and years of practice before I was closer to the second scenario.

Patients expect certain things from their veterinarian, and frequently those expectations are different from those the doctor needs to meet to make a correct diagnosis. A good example of this was told by TSH. He talks about a time in the hills of Jamaica, where a team from his medical school had a project. They were fourth-year medical students, and presumably more knowledgeable than the public health nurse that served this region. These people of the village attached magical significance to the stethoscope, and their term for the application of the stethoscope to their various body parts was "sounding." If you were looking at their eye, they wanted you to sound it, and the same for a joint or skin lesion. If you neglected this part of the exam, they would remind you to sound them, and if you refused or totally forgot, they felt less confident of your abilities and were disappointed in their encounter with you.

Sounding was an important part of reassuring those Jamaican patients, part of reassurance therapy for them. The several components of reassurance therapy comprise listening to the client's complaint, asking questions to demonstrate that you are hearing them, examining the patient with special attention given to the affected body part, and then delivering an opinion. Remember that part of reassurance therapy is examination. You may have the diagnosis nailed from the lab test or the patient's history, but they want you to examine the affected part anyway. So the laying on of hands, the examination, the sounding, if you will, even if you don't need to do it for your purposes, reassures and satisfies the patient.

Reassurance Therapy

Six steps:
1. Elicit detailed description of symptom
2. Elicit affective meaning of the symptom
3. Examine patient
4. Make a diagnosis
5. Explain symptom to client
6. Reassure the client

Sounding reassured Jamaican patients and also taught me the importance of reassuring clients while doing the correct thing medically.

Another expectation: clients expect you to "look" like a doctor. Traditionally this means wearing a white coat, a powerful symbol of being a physician. It means conservative dress for women and men. Fred Plum, MD, a renowned neurologist, explained the need to look like a doctor in the patient's eyes by invoking the concept of the spectrum of egocentricity (orientation to yourself) to eccentricity (orientation to others) that carries over well to our field. The wilder and more casual your dress, the more tattoos or body piercings you display, the more unruly your hair or your beard, the more you seem oriented to yourself, and indeed you are and you may be proud of it. But clients want you to be oriented to *them and their pet*, not to yourself, and this includes looking the traditional part of the doctor in dress and demeanor. So what's your orientation and whom are you trying to please? What does your appearance communicate about you? Are you trying to tell the world how wild and free you are, how unique you are, what an individual you are, all things most clients have no interest in? Or are you telling your clients that you care about their pets, and you realize the importance of looking the part so they have confidence in your abilities as a doctor? For an opposing view, a recent article in the *Wall Street Journal* discusses the emerging view that lab coats, ties, and anything with sleeves possibly spreads infection. This contention is under study, and as the article discusses, many doctors feel the white coat is very important.[1] Whether the

---

1   Rebecca Smith, "Nothing to Sneeze At: Doctors' Neckties Seen As Flu Risk," *Wall Street Journal*, 26 July 2009: 1.

white coat disappears in certain settings or not, you should present a dignified and conservative appearance when you are seeing patients.

Whatever you wear, keep in mind that the first impression a patient gains is crucial. You want it to be a good one, and you only get one chance. You want that impression made on your ability, not on what you look like.

Business Writing

Keep it short, very short, and this involves more organization and thought than a brain dump, but your reader will appreciate it. Everyone is busy, and very few will read with care any communication longer than a page or a page and a half. If your writing is any longer than this, the reader takes in only 10 percent of what you write. If it has to be long, get your main points in early. If you're writing a letter to a referring veterinarian, get to the diagnosis and treatment plan quickly—those are the main points of interest to that particular reader. You may be proud of the great exam you did and all the tests you ordered, but all that means little to the average harried practitioner who has a million things on his desk and wants only the essentials from you.

Use the features of your word processor. Break up the text into small paragraphs since a long block of text is daunting. Use the *bold* feature and bullet points to organize your text and make the reading easier. Think about how to make the letter easy for the reader, and after a while, it will be second nature.

Meetings

Meetings can and do waste a lot of time, but when they're needed and run effectively, they can produce positive outcomes. Meet only:

1. When the group needs to make a decision and more than one person is needed to provide expertise or information
2. When you must decide between several acceptable solutions and each solution has its advocates
3. When the personal presence of several people is essential to the meeting's objectives

If the meeting can be reduced to a handout and no decisions need to be made, send that out and cancel the meeting.

If you lead the meeting, make sure the agenda is correct. A good agenda should include:

1. Day, time, and place of the meeting. Many people just grab the agenda on the way out the door and can't remember the time or meeting place
2. The names of those attending
3. The objectives of the meeting
4. The topics for discussion, the person leading off the discussion, and a time limit for each topic

The agenda and any related reading material should arrive on the desk of each participant ideally a week ahead of the meeting. Everyone is busy, and a thick packet of paper a day or two ahead of a meeting only frustrates your attendees, who may simply be unable to review a lot of material on short notice.

As the leader of the meeting, you should be sure that the time limit for each topic is reasonable, and you should ruthlessly enforce that time limit. When you are the leader, you are the servant of the group, and one huge job is to respect the time of your participants. You do this by starting on time and, most of all, ending on time. Most meetings are periodic, and you will be chairing these meetings for several years. If you start on time, the latecomers will learn this and begin arriving for the beginning. If you end on time consistently, your attendees will appreciate this, making you a rare commodity. To stay on track, make sure to wind up discussions by keeping each topic on schedule. There are always those who like to hear themselves speak, and frequently just repeat what someone else has just said. Learn how to nicely cut them off and focus on a vote or whatever it takes to keep on schedule. As you gain a reputation for timeliness, your group will learn how to behave and will know that they have to help keep to the time limits. You'll be amazed at the gratitude you engender simply by ending a meeting on time consistently.

Public Speaking

Books and seminars address this topic in more detail than we can in this book, but a few details should help.

- First, plan your talk, whether it's a discussion at a meeting, a scientific presentation, or a speech to the public.
- Know your audience and tailor your remarks appropriately.
- Discuss between two and four major topics, each with two to four subheadings.
- Any more than these, and you have lost your audience. Provide a road map at the beginning and summarize as you go along, reminding the audience where you are.

- Use slides and other visuals only for clarity and emphasis. Don't clutter up a slide. Each slide should have only three or four easily read points. How often have you heard a mumbled apology from the podium, "I know this is a busy slide, but . . ." What the speaker means is, "I was too lazy to make a slide that effectively shows my point, so I'm using one that I already had, and now that I'm up here, I wish I had done better."
- Look at the audience, not the slide. You are speaking to people, not a screen.
- Remember that your words are only 7 percent of your message, as with any full-channel, face-to-face communication, and the remaining 93 percent comes from voice inflection and body language—especially eye contact. Rehearse if at all possible. If this is an important speech, rehearse with a coach. Outline your talk, and speak from that. Do not read a speech.

Good speakers have:

1. **Authority** - This means your posture, your personal appearance, and your voice.
2. **Audience awareness** - Make eye contact with a variety of people. Use pauses effectively.
3. **Energy** - Use gestures, and express yourself with body language and your face. Don't sway or nervously twitch.
4. **Road maps and summaries** - Unless the audience has a handout, they don't know your talk as you know it. Let them know ahead of time the major topics, remembering that audiences can take in three, at most four, points in a spoken presentation.

Summarize where you have been and where you are going so the audience can stick with you.

The audience is rooting for you. They fear failure on your part just as you do. They fear getting lost in the talk, hence the need for road maps and summaries. They also fear boredom, so put some energy into your talk and make it the best you can.

Chapter 5: Organizational Behavior

This is the business person's "OB," and it deals with the complexities of human behavior within organizations. When I commiserate with veterinarians, we all agree that managing the office and employees is the worst part of practicing medicine. Indeed, across most businesses, leaders agree with this assessment. This is because it is truly troublesome in every business, and especially for veterinarians, because many of us have had no preparation or training in this area. You are not immune if you work for a big organization with staff to handle human resources. You will still be confronted with interpersonal problems, bickering, and self-interested requests.

If you're solo, you not only have to deal with employees, but you also have to deal with many more issues because you can't hire a human resources staffer. You may have an office manager, but you will still hear about the problems. If you are in group practice, the employees' problems will still reach you, but not as directly. However, you will face issues unknown to solo practitioners—the problems of living with a bunch of veterinarians.

Employees

Unless you are a solo veterinarian and have only a very limited staff, your employees will make or break your practice. You can be a great vet, but if patients get turned off by your appointment process or can never get an answer back from your staff when they call with problems, you will lose them. You will also get poor ratings when those client satisfaction surveys go out. Why? Because clients judge you by the entire experience with your office, not just by your medical skills. They have no way to judge your professional ability, so they use surrogate measures, and most of these involve your staff and office setup.

At the highest level, you have to model proper behavior. Eventually, your staff will reflect your behavior and attitudes. If you don't care about the ease of getting appointments, neither will your staff. If you don't care to answer clients' questions in a timely manner, neither will your staff. If they see that you don't care, neither will they, and they will do what suits them, not the patient or client. You can't just issue orders but never follow up with reports or inspections; staff will learn that about you as well. They will let you rant and rave about what you want and will go on doing what they want because they know you won't follow up. The culture of an office, a research lab, or an academic department is set from the top. In time, you will get what you model and demonstrate what you care about. So start with yourself.

Culture and More Culture

By starting with your own attitudes and modeling these for staff, you are setting the culture for your practice or area within your organization. In the best of instances, you joined an organization that had the right culture and all you have to do is fit in and do your part. In the worst, the overall culture is bad and you have to struggle to establish yours in your section or individual area. This is much harder, but the principles are the same.

Set the tone. You are not just the manager, you're the leader. Leaders set the vision and tone, while managers make sure these are followed. You are both the leader and the manager, so you have double responsibilities.

Make your policies clear and communicate them to all the staff, not just the managers. Examine your organization's mission statement, if there is one. Adopt a mission statement for your area even if it seems a bit hokey. If you construct a mission statement, do so with the help of your staff. This gives them a sense of ownership in that mission, so that it's a joint undertaking, not a set of commands from above. In this way, you will increase your success rate in setting a good culture. Such a statement should be concise and easy to read, and it should motivate employees to take good care of patients and provide a setting that creates a "wow" from everyone who enters your doors.

You can't just model behavior; you have to let your staff know that you expect the same attitudes and treatment of patients that you model for them. Remember, you're the boss, not a coworker and underling the way you were when you were a trainee. Making the transition from colleague to boss is difficult for all levels of new managers across all industries. You, like many others in the corporate world, have no idea of the rules or skills of being a manager and will flounder. Erin White wrote of these issues in a *Wall Street Journal* article in November 2005.[1] She pointed out the common mistakes made by new managers:

1. Wanting to stay pals with your former peers. This is especially true of those who stay in the same academic setting or practice where they trained.
2. Asserting your new authority too harshly and coming down too hard on former peers.
3. Not giving a problem employee honest feedback so you can avoid conflict.
4. Wanting to keep doing the work yourself rather than developing your employees' skills.

Some of the core skills you need to learn are: coaching, leading, disciplining, giving feedback, and resolving conflicts. Commonly, only the largest organizations provide training to new managers. White's article said, "Among the worst offenders are organizations filled with professionals, such as lawyers, doctors and journalists, who consider themselves masters of their craft first and managers second."

You may think to yourself that you only wanted to be a veterinarian—not a manager. Well, you're a manager whether you want to be or not. You will have an area in which you practice or conduct your research. Employees in that area will consider you their boss and bring their problems to you, whether you want them or not. We can assure you, you want satisfied employees, if only for your own peace of mind.

---

[1] Erin White, "Learning to be the Boss," *Wall Street Journal*, 21 Nov. 2005: B1.

Employee Satisfaction

The following ten factors influence employee satisfaction, listed in order of importance:

1. Career opportunities
2. Learning new skills
3. Promotion
4. Pay
5. Responsibility
6. Autonomy
7. Personal sense of satisfaction
8. Praise
9. Job security
10. Respect

As you can see, you can influence some of these by your behavior as manager.

You may or may not control salaries when you are new to a practice, but you can provide feedback to those who do. Career opportunities and promotions are limited in a veterinary office. If you're a nurse or a technician, you will remain so. Most offices do not have a career ladder outlined for those at lower levels. So what can you do? Emphasize the areas you can help with, such as learning new skills and giving responsibility and autonomy, within reason and ethical bounds. You can praise people and show respect, giving them a personal sense of satisfaction. By your awareness of these issues, you can do your part in keeping your staff as satisfied as possible.

The two factors that influence employee dissatisfaction are personal conflicts with other employees, an area where you can intervene if appropriate, and personal life factors outside the office. You cannot control someone's personal life, nor should you try. You may be tempted to act as a counselor (and it may not be possible or even humane to avoid hearing about someone's travails at home), but you should not embroil yourself deeply in domestic problems. Not only do you cross the line from boss to friend, but you're probably not qualified in this area.

Only lately have I learned, slowly and painfully, the following lesson: Stay out of the crossfire. If two people are having a conflict and you're just sure you can help out by jumping in with your thoughts on a resolution, watch it. You're likely not aware of all the issues, and the most likely outcome of your interference is both parties being angry at you and turning on you. This is true for friends and family as well as work situations.

Another lesson—there are *always* two sides to every story. You may hear one side and be perfectly convinced that person is in the right, but we guarantee you the other side has a story as well. Before you make a judgment, be sure you've heard the other side.

Fellow Doctors

If you're solo, you can skip this section or read on to realize one advantage of your type of practice: not having to deal with veterinary partners. Believe it or not, vets are people, human beings just like everyone else. The unspoken message given to veterinarians is that we're just a little bit special, and that certain rules don't apply to us. The main theme of this book is that our training misled us into believing that we are exempt from the principles of business and management and therefore don't need to bother with such details. But there are other myths out there:

Veterinarians are wonderful people. They sacrificed their early years by their devotion to their studies, and all they want is the best for you (patients, colleagues, fellow veterinarians, whomever) and they don't care about themselves or their own welfare.

Veterinarians deserve a break. They don't have to be bound by the normal rules governing interpersonal relationships. They can abuse staff, be rude to nurses in the hospital, and say what they want at cocktail parties.

Veterinarians know it all. Because they studied hard to learn anatomy and other subjects, they know a lot about politics, investing, managing a complex business like a hospital, the environment, and just about anything else. You can believe whatever they say.

Veterinarians never lie or manipulate the truth. Society should grant them privileges so they can never be sued for something they say because, after all, they would never harm someone by misrepresenting an issue.

Veterinarians want only the best for their patients and nothing for themselves. Their only interest in life is high-quality care for their patients. For example, they would never not refer clients to a specialist for a new procedure because of turf interests or because they would lose patients. Instead they're only interested in patients' welfare.

If you've been paying attention during your years of training, you know these are not always true. You've seen the power struggles in academia and heard the petty things professors say about those at other institutions, but how does this apply to your practice life?

First, as always, look to yourself. Make sure you haven't given into those "rules." Behave like a human being, not the stereotypical veterinarian. Be polite. Don't act like you know everything, and tell the truth. Know whether your advocacy for a given issue is truly for patient care or not.

Keep an open mind as you get to know your colleagues, and don't assume that they're saints. In the same respect, don't assume they're your enemy either. You will find that most veterinarians are like most other people—reasonable, fairly nice, interested in doing their jobs to the best of their ability and getting home to relax and be with their families. However, there are a few types of veterinarians you need to look out for:

Troublemaker

Is someone always agitating against the powers that be in the group, constantly complaining about how unfair certain things are? Are they pulling aside vets to bring up issues in whispered hallway conversations or complaining about relatively minor issues at meetings?

Some vets aren't happy unless they're stirring up trouble. To do so, they create issues that aren't important so they can do the aforementioned and get whatever satisfaction this brings to them. Their complaints may sound perfectly justified, and you may be sucked into supporting them, but watch out. Group harmony is a precarious luxury, and each individual has to sacrifice something to the interests of the group.

Some people are optimizers and feel that every detail should be perfect, no matter how small or irrelevant that detail is to the big picture. Some are "satisfiers," happy to get the important things right but they realize that the time, effort, and expense of making everything totally right make optimizing impractical. So some complaining is done by the optimizers and some is done by troublemakers—either way, the group suffers. A number of complaints are legitimate and changes need to be made, so, as always, use good judgment and be aware if the same person is always the complainer.

You can't be a member of a group yet have your way on every issue. So you should be careful, especially in your first few years, that you don't become an unwitting ally for the troublemaking vet. If an optimizer latches on to you, learn how to gently disengage and point out the big picture. Agree that in an ideal world, they are correct, but alas, the world is not ideal.

Abuser

Veterinarians who abuse hospital or office staff used to be tolerated, or at least ignored by the power structure. No more. Such doctors are frequently excellent clinicians and have positions of power or influence, making it harder for others in power to intervene. Dr. Kent Neff has written an excellent chapter in his book *Enhancing Physician Performance*, for the American College of Physician Executives, on this subject.[2] He gives examples of disruptive behavior:

---

2   Kent Neff, "Understanding and Managing Physicians with Disruptive Behavior," in Scott Ransom et al (editors), *Enhancing Physician Performance: Advanced*

- Profane or disrespectful language
- Demeaning behavior, i.e., referring to hospital staff as "stupid"
- Sexual comments or innuendo
- Inappropriate touching, sexual or otherwise
- Racial or ethnically oriented jokes (i.e. jokes made at the expense of others)
- Outbursts of anger
- Throwing instruments or charts (i.e., temper tantrums)
- Criticizing hospital staff in front of patients or other staff
- Negative comments about another physician's care
- Boundary violations with staff or patients
- Comments that undermine a patient's trust in a physician or hospital
- Inappropriate chart notes
- Unethical or dishonest behavior
- Failure to respond to repeated calls
- Poor response to corrective action

When you are new to a group, you lack the power or standing to deal with such doctors. You need only to recognize this behavior as abnormal, discreetly report it to your mentor or group leader, then avoid the crossfire. If your leaders fail to address the problem, harass them and insist on corrective action. There are legal issues involved, and these can embroil the entire group, affecting you in a negative way even though you are minding your own business. Early intervention is the key.

Principles of Medical Management. American College of Physician Executives: 2000.

Incompetent

Unfortunately, the strict standards for admission to veterinary school and training don't always exclude those who later prove to be inadequate to the job of patient care, and you may encounter degrees of incompetence in colleagues in your group or on your hospital staff. Some doctors just don't have it; others do well with the more basic aspects of their specialty but aren't up to handling complicated problems. Knowing limits is important. A doctor who knows his or her limitations and refers problems to others accordingly can have a lifetime of successful practice.

Some vets do well with routine operations but can't handle the harder ones. Others do well with the outpatient practice but mishandle complicated patients. If you're early in your group practice career, you may notice such vets by seeing their problems. The more established members of the group may be more isolated because they see only their own patients and don't have the opportunity to see the problems. More likely, these vets recognize the problem but are turning a blind eye because it is easier than confronting the issue.

What should you do? You owe it to your group's patients and the long-term reputation of the group to do something, even if you're so new to the group that you have no power. If you have attached yourself to a mentor or are particularly close to a partner, talk to that vet. You will need concrete examples of poor or potentially dangerous outcomes. Innuendo and vague feelings are not sufficient. You're embarking down a path with career-threatening outcomes to established veterinarians.

Lawsuits could result, and you need to be very careful. At this stage of your career, your obligation ends with turning the problem over to a more senior partner in the group. We will discuss their duties in a later section.

If you've reported a legitimate problem, nothing is done, and problems continue, you've learned something about your group, and you need to decide if such a group is suitable for you. If you've noticed a problem vet, others in the community will also. If you're in a group that tolerates marginal veterinarians, your reputation will suffer over time. If you conclude that your group tolerates marginal or incompetent veterinarians for whatever reason, you should leave before your personal reputation begins to suffer. You can be sure that other vets in your community know the same thing you do, and they will be watching you to see if you fit in and accept such conditions or leave. Be careful and be sure of your grounds, but make a move if you have to.

Greedy

Does one of your group order more tests than anyone else, or operate consistently in borderline situations? Does such a veterinarian refer to patients only in terms of money, of the potential income of a given type of patient? Does this vet refuse to see pets that do not generate much money? Over time, do you get a feeling that finances, not compassion, rule a partner's thoughts and actions?

Believe it or not, some people entered veterinary medicine only because of the financial advantages of being a doctor. They hid their true ambitions during the training years, and may have paid more attention to their moonlighting jobs than their education. The truth comes out when they begin practice. The competence level of such vets can range from marginal (a particularly bad combination) to excellent. The consistent feature is that their decisions on testing or operating are ruled not by concern for the patient but for their own pocketbook.

The most important reason to avoid over-testing and marginally indicated surgery is your obligation to the patient. Many tests and all surgical procedures have some degree of risk. Subjecting a patient to risk of problems is reasonable when there is proper indication. If your patient suffers a complication from a procedure that wasn't necessary in the first place, you have wronged that pet. It simply isn't right to harm animals, especially when you have taken an oath to do the opposite.

Moreover, you have created a potential legal nightmare. Unhappy clients seek other opinions, causing double jeopardy for you, the risk of a malpractice suit, and a nail in the coffin of your reputation.

Veterinarians with good reputations get more patients and are well regarded in the community. Regard in the community leads to a better social life for your family and leadership positions for you, if you want them. If a patient with a bad outcome from your appropriate treatment seeks a second opinion, the new doctor will assure that patient of your competence and stature, helping to avoid an unnecessary lawsuit. Attorneys become aware of who's who in the veterinary community as well. They would be less likely to take on an icon in the community than a pariah. (Of course, there are some desperate lawyers who will take on anything and anyone, but the good ones, believe it or not, exercise some judgment about the people they sue.)

So avoid greedy behavior and don't allow it in your practice, even if it means changing practices or firing a colleague.

Lazy

Veterinarians work hard. They have to study harder than most in college to gain admission to veterinary school, then work even harder through veterinary education and training. Therefore, every vet will work hard when he or she begins practice, correct?

Not always. Just as there are many different personalities in veterinary medicine, there are also many different types of work ethic. Moreover, when veterinarians make the transition from a fixed salary to private practice, some have trouble. The difference: a fixed salary vs. fee-for-service in private practice. In the real world of fee-for-service, your productivity determines your income. Magically enough, the financial incentive of greater income for seeing more patients leads to seeing more patients and working harder. All of a sudden, that same vet can see patients the day after his night on call. The paperwork can be done after hours or between patients, or delegated. In this scenario, most veterinarians become more productive.

It's obvious that vets respond to financial incentives. But what happens if income is less directly tied to work? What happens to veterinarians in private practice who work only on a fixed salary? I can guarantee you that leaders of such groups deal with vets who don't want to do their share. They can't be located when that emergency call comes in. They shift that late afternoon patient to the young vet. They take a long lunch or coffee break. They only want to see a set number of patients a day. Their colleagues recognize this behavior for what it is, and complaints go to the leader. Some leaders tackle such problems head-on; others just make more rules. Remember, it's painful to fire a doctor, so some groups will tolerate behavior like this.

What if the veterinarian has independent money? Even in a group that has income directly tied to work, lazy behavior can result. A group we know once hired a young doctor who said all the right things during the interview process. The group hired him, and after they hired him, they found out that his father was wealthy and shared a lot of his money with his son. The result after a few years was a three-day workweek for that doctor. No amount of encouragement, both nice and not so nice, could induce him to work harder.

The group was totally unable to influence his behavior. They didn't fire him, because they liked him and he did good work, albeit less than they wanted. From the group's perspective, he was occupying a slot that should have been producing a certain amount of income and contribution to overhead, and his reduced production penalized the group by forcing them to pay more overhead. From his perspective, the group was robbing him of his income by taking a bigger percentage of his production for overhead. Eventually he left that group for another.

So what should the young vet do? Such lazy senior vets will soon declare themselves to you by their behavior, and you'll come to know them. "I have to go to a meeting; will you see this patient for me?" Or from the staff, "We can't find Doctor X, will you see this patient? She really needs to be seen now." Early on, your hands are tied since you want to be well regarded by the group, and you'll just work a little harder. You don't have much recourse unless you have a mentor to whom you can complain. When you come to a more senior position and you're interviewing young vets, you might ask a few questions to elicit knowledge of the prospect's financial situation. From the group's perspective, a new vet with a family and debt will magically produce someone who works hard, at least in a group like ours.

Sociopath

Whether you call them sociopaths, psychopaths, or white-collar psychopaths, they exist in all of society, including veterinary medicine. They are glib and charming, always saying the right thing. Clients love them and allow them to do whatever they want to their patients. They ingratiate themselves to their superiors in the administrative food chain while demeaning those below them. They advance through the ranks rapidly, often leaping over unsuspecting colleagues and immediate superiors.

They have no conscience and don't care what happens to others. Nothing is ever their fault and they do no wrong. They are frequently paranoid and grandiose. If you suspect you're dealing with one of these types of people, watch out. They will squash you if you get in their way.

> **REFERENCES ON SOCIOPATHS:**
>
> Two good books:
>
> *Without Conscience: The Disturbing World of the Psychopaths Among Us* by Robert Hare (The Guilford Press: 1999)
>
> *The Sociopath Next Door* by Martha Stout (Broadway: 2006)

If you think you may have a sociopath as a colleague or superior, be very careful before making this judgment; it's a devastating diagnosis. Once you label someone a sociopath, by definition, you can never trust what they say, since lying is second nature to them. An innocent person mislabeled a sociopath can never successfully defend himself because no defense can be believed. So gather your evidence. Talk to trusted colleagues, perhaps a mental-health professional, and be sure of your facts and interpretations.

If you are sure of the diagnosis, proceed carefully. Since this is a character disorder and can never be remedied, the best option is for someone to leave—either that person or you. Yet another option is relentless monitoring by someone who has true authority over the sociopath and is willing to exert it. Be aware that a characteristic of sociopaths is their ingratiating behavior to those in charge. They may have been to the dean or chairman before you, complaining about you and poisoning your superiors against you when you come with legitimate complaints. If they occupy a position of power, those with power over them can be charmed, making it dangerous for those below to make headway. If you make a move to dislodge such a person, be sure of your success before undertaking this option. The more junior you are, the less your chance of success in deposing a superior and the more you should consider leaving and keeping your name and reputation from being ensnared with that of the sociopath. Whatever you do, don't just stay and put up with a colleague's sociopathic behavior. You will be damaged eventually.

Impaired Doctor

In veterinary medicine we have access to addictive drugs. Whatever the reason, whether it's genetics, stress, or access, some vets are impaired by addiction to alcohol or drugs.

Psychiatrists look on addiction as a chronic disease with remissions and relapses, and they have fashioned rehabilitation programs aimed at professionals. A lingering concept in many minds, and perhaps of those who are addicted, is that a character flaw or defect produces addiction. Whatever the thought process is, vets often hide their addiction, and eventually their behavior—not their own confession or admission—gives them away.

If you are addicted or are prone to addiction, get help as soon as possible. There are many programs that deal with veterinarians in total confidentiality, hoping to prevent suicide and other problems. State boards and other regulatory bodies look with favor on self-admission of problems and proactive therapy in the appropriate program. If it takes a DUI or other legal situation to bring your problem to light, they will mandate not only treatment, but also random testing to be sure you're clean. Because of this, not many addicted veterinarians take the self-admission route. It usually takes a disaster to bring the problem to the attention of those who can mandate treatment.

If you're new to a group and witness behavior signaling addiction, your responsibility is to report that to the group's leader. If it's not handled appropriately, you have learned something negative about your group. If your leadership addresses the problem in correct fashion, you have learned something else. If you're the group's leader, more on this later, but these problems can't be ignored.

What if your only partner is addicted? As much as you might hope this will go away, it won't. Furthermore, you have definite moral, legal, and ethical responsibilities once you're sure of such a situation. You must be sure the patients are protected. You can't handle this by yourself. Seek professional help to deal with this. You will need the advice of a mental-health professional in dealing with the personal problem and a lawyer on the potential legal problem. If the problem continues untreated and you've done all you can without finding a solution, you may need to leave the practice. The absolute worst approach is to put your head in the sand and soldier on. If you do not address the problem early, disaster in some form will eventually come.

Fortunately, most veterinarians do not fall into any of the aforementioned categories. Your greatest risk in joining a group is that you simply don't like some of your colleagues, and you can live with this. If you're unlucky and you encounter some of the problems discussed in this chapter, recognize that there is a problem, diagnose it carefully and accurately, and then deal with it.

Chapter 6: Marketing

You may be thinking, *Marketing! I don't need to advertise.* Most veterinarians are conservative, cheap, and clueless and hate the thought of advertising (and confuse it with marketing). Therefore, their eyes glaze over at the mention of either one. Marketing, properly understood and executed, should be a daily activity for vets. Advertising is totally distinct from marketing and necessary in only a few specialties.

Marketing is the process of finding out what your customers want, designing a product to fulfill their desires, and letting them know you have done so. Applied to veterinary medicine, it's the process of finding out what your patients or referring veterinarians want, creating a service to meet that want, and letting them know it's available. Let's look at some general aspects of marketing as applied to any business, and apply the principles to a veterinary practice.

Place

The physical setting should be dignified, conservative, and clean. It should connote caring and effectiveness. As the day goes on, do your exam floors accumulate hair, bits of alcohol sponges, and other debris? Do you pick them up, thereby setting a good example for your staff? Make sure the same is done for your check-in area and hallway. How does your office furniture look? Have you let things get old and worn? Do you need new paint or wallpaper for the walls or the outside of your building?

People

Office staff—front, back, and technical—should look professional in their dress and appearance. They should exude care and friendliness. Do not allow them to sit behind a closed glass partition, looking up reluctantly every now and then. You should have an open greeting space, with a welcoming air and a smiling face for each patient to see.

Equipment

Diagnostic equipment should look new or at least neat and clean. Exam rooms should look neat and tidy as well.

Access

The service is located at convenient locations at times that suit the consumer and with little waiting. How long do your patients and clients wait to see you? What do you do when you get behind? Some vets just plow ahead and gut it out while others take a more proactive approach. Queue management is a science in itself, well studied by Disney and other companies. Patients understand that veterinarians get behind, but they want to know so they can plan their time. Uncertainty is the problem. If you're running late, let the patients know about how long it will be. They also want to know why you're late that day. If your staff keeps them posted about when and why, giving them a realistic estimate of when they will be seen and finished, they will be in a much better mood when you do get to them.

Communication

You should have brochures that explain the common conditions you treat, written in lay language. There are many companies that make them, and the clients appreciate them. You should send clients out with their new treatment plan written clearly; most clients simply will not remember your plan.

Competence

Employees must possess the required skill and knowledge. It is difficult for a client to know that you or your staff are competent for sure, hence these other measures, but it's easy to tell when your staff are incompetent or unskilled.

Courtesy

Employees are friendly, respectful, and considerate.

Responsiveness

Employees respond quickly and creatively.

Understanding/Knowing

Employees make the effort to understand the client's needs and provide individual attention.

Clearly, there is more to satisfying the client and the patient than curing or managing their disease. In these days, more and more hospitals send out patient satisfaction surveys and judge your service by the results. You will get better scores when you follow these precepts.

Business academicians have thoroughly studied the best managed-service companies. Here's what it takes:

1. A history of top management commitment to quality: If your staff doesn't see you committed to quality and if you don't demand it from them, you won't get it.
2. Setting high standards
3. Systems for monitoring service performance: You can do this by comparison shopping, ghost shopping, and providing surveys and suggestion forms in the office.
4. Satisfying employees as well as the customers:

Disney and other companies spend weeks training their new employees and keep them trained as well. What do you do? Do you make employee happiness part of your job?

Veterinary Marketing

With these general principles in mind, let's examine veterinary marketing in more detail.

THE CLIENT

Dr. Harbin's marketing professor encouraged a game called Let's Go Shopping. Put yourself in the shoes of your client and look at things from their perspective. Have a friend call your office. How long did it take to get to a human being? What was the tone of the receptionist, and how long is the wait to get an appointment with you? Do you offer an introductory brochure and map? Do you have good information on your website that the office referred to you? Did they offer to email you directions to the office?

Come in to your office early one day and look at the tangible aspects. Is it clean and attractive? Do you have up-to-date reading material? Are your payment and fee policies clear? Are your exam rooms neat? Look again at the end of the day. Are they just as clean for the last patient as they were for the first?

How about the employees? Are they friendly and concerned, and dressed professionally? Do they keep their personal concerns out of the clients' earshot?

Ask some of your employees their impression of the aforementioned issues. When they know you are interested, they can tell you things that clients tell them, things they keep to themselves until they see you care about them.

Don't stop with a one-time Let's Go Shopping. You should periodically survey your clients with a formal, written instrument that they mail back to you or to whomever you hire to survey them. You can also now have an automatically generated survey that is e-mailed or texted to them after their visit. By so doing, you make clients feel that you are concerned about their opinion and you pick up on problems before they become major. If you're not motivated to do a survey, you should do one anyway; it can give you invaluable information about your practice.

Referral Sources

Remember that the best orientation is the market orientation, in which you are attuned to the needs and desires of your market and deliver accordingly. You need to know these factors for those who send you patients. Whoever refers to you wants the process to be quick and easy, with minimal time arranging the visit. They want quality care for their patient and they want owners to come back singing your praises. This applies more to a referral hospital as opposed to a general practice hospital.

If you're new in practice, how do you find these sources in the first place? Of course, it differs for every specialty and practice situation. Even if you're joining a group, you need to consider your sources. At the very least, send out an announcement, but be aware of what happens to these when they land on the desk of a busy doctor. A quick glance, a mental note of "That's nice," and into the trash, soon forgotten. Remember that the words of any given message constitute a small portion of the overall message, and the rest comes from personal factors. A formal announcement, while traditional and necessary, is a pale substitute for a personal visit. Nothing substitutes for a face-to-face meeting when you want maximum impact.

You should survey your referral sources just as you do your clients. You will find out any bottlenecks and frustrations encountered in getting patients to you and will be able to correct them.

PRACTICAL TIPS FOR REFERRAL SOURCES:
- Keep them supplied with maps and brochures.
- Give a small, tasteful gift during the holidays.
- Track referrals and know who is slacking off.
- Know the communication desires of each doctor.
- Know who wants you to treat, and who wants you just to diagnose and send back.
- Send periodic satisfaction surveys.

As you track referrals, you will find some who keep sending you patients and others who either totally quit or diminish their volume. You should find out why, and many times your survey will not reveal the problem. You will need to visit or call yourself. You may find that one of your staff angered one of the doctor's staff members, or that your behavior is the problem. Whatever it is, knowing it will allow you a chance to fix it. When you treat referral sources as one of your target markets, you will be rewarded with a busier practice.

Employees

Not all your markets are external, and employees represent an internal market to which you should orient yourself. Studies of the leading service companies show that they have happy and well-trained employees. Remember that because of a patient's inability to measure your services directly, they use employees as well as the other tangible factors to judge your quality.

You probably like it when your clients thank you for what you have done for them, even when you know you did no different or better than one of your colleagues. You should thank your staff when they do their jobs, even when you know they were just doing what they should have been doing. Do you have lunch brought in for no special occasion? Do you keep track of birthdays and give appropriate gifts both then and during the holidays? Reread the section in chapter five on employee satisfaction to note the ways you can make employees happy without giving them a raise.

What about training? Do you throw employees to the wolves by putting them on your front desk or in your clinic with no orientation? Do you have formal ways of getting them trained? Some pay a bonus when a technician passes the training course sponsored by the official, academy-affiliated technician organization. Our pay scales are different for those who are certified and those who aren't. The doctors give occasional lectures at group-sponsored lunch meetings, and we show interesting findings to the technicians as we go along.

Ongoing training ranks just as high as initial training. Do you pay for your staff to go to meetings? Our group does by providing a yearly allowance for continuing education. Do you have good internal communications? The "CEO disease" refers to those at the top who are out of touch with the troops. Do you mix and mingle with the staff, talk to them, and keep aware of their issues? Do you walk around areas you don't usually frequent, just so the staff knows you might pop up anytime? It keeps them on their toes and off the Internet. A well-trained staff impresses clients and makes your life immeasurably easier. Keep employees in mind as your third market.

Internet

Social networking has assumed importance in recent years. LinkedIn, Facebook, and Twitter have become avenues for communicating with clients and perhaps referral sources. Also be sure to monitor your Internet presence on different sites where people can leave comments about your service. The ways to use social networking to market and enhance a practice change almost weekly, and the details are beyond the scope of this book. Nevertheless, this area is important. The younger you are, the more familiar you are with the Internet; older vets need to spend time in this area, probably with professional help.

Chapter 7: Economics

The intricate mathematical relationships between price, demand, and supply don't apply well in veterinary medicine. The economically correct way to think about costs, however, does apply to decisions made in veterinary practice.

Cost Analysis

We all make financial decisions, trying to consider the costs involved in making the most rational use of our time and money. Let's say you wanted to build a new or satellite office. A year ago you paid an architect $5,000 for plans and then changed your mind. You resurrect the plans, and they're still good. You have two staffers with you all the time at a cost of $400 a day. It will cost you $50,000 to build out the space and an extra $10,000 a year in rent. But you will be busier in this space, and you will collect $500 a week more than you would at your current space.

So let's look at one year. The table lists all the costs:

All costs for first year of satellite office:
Plans: $5,000   Build-out: $50,000
Rent: $10,000   Staff: $20,000 (400 x 50)
Total Cost: $85,000

With this analysis, the project is a loser and should not be pursued. As you may have guessed, the analysis is incorrect. You would have flunked this portion of the microeconomics exam by making the assumptions in the table. Economists define different types of costs, some of which should not enter an analysis like the one we provided:

Sunk Costs

These are costs that have been spent no matter what and are already done. They do not enter into a forward-looking analysis. In this example, the $5,000 for the plans is a sunk cost. You already have spent those dollars and will never recover them.

Committed Costs

These are costs that you would have to spend in the future, no matter what. The staff salaries are committed costs and would have to be paid regardless of your going ahead with this project. These costs are not part of this analysis unless you plan to keep this new satellite staffed even if you're not present. If you do, and depending on the level of staffing, the costs should be considered.

Relevant Costs

These are also called incremental costs, and are defined as costs that would change as a result of the new project. These are also the costs that are properly included in the analysis here. You also have to think of relevant costs for a given period. Since the space will be used for much longer than one year, you should not assign all the build-out costs to the first year, but only a reasonable portion.

Since this is a long-term project, let's recast the table to the liking of an economist. We assume a ten-year project, so the build-out will be spread over that period.

> Correct cost analysis of satellite office:
>
> Plans: $5,000 sunk cost, not part of analysis
>
> Build-Out: $50,000 for ten-year project, only $5,000 relevant
>
> Rent: $10,000, a relevant cost and should be considered
>
> Staff: $20,000 committed cost, not part of analysis
>
> Total relevant cost: $15,000 or more if both facilities are to be fully staffed.

Now this compares favorably to the $25,000 in extra income.

Opportunity Cost

There's one more cost to be considered: opportunity cost. This is a cost that is somewhat harder to get your head around. Opportunity cost is the value of a resource in its best alternative use. If you have to borrow the $50,000 for the build-out and spend $10,000 in rent, what else could you do with $60,000? Invest it and make $10,000 for each of the next ten years? Not likely, and if you could, you're in the wrong profession, at least from a purely financial standpoint. An economist would insist that you consider opportunity cost. If you could use a resource in a different way and make more, you should consider the alternative, unless you had other strategic reasons to stick to your first choice.

What did it cost you to go to school and undergo your training for all those years? If you add up the tuition and living costs and use that as a total, you ignore your opportunity costs. If you had not been in training, you would have been working. So your salary for those years should be added to your direct costs of tuition, etc. Then you have a true picture of all your costs for your education.

This is a highly simplified cost analysis, but it makes the point. Consider only the relevant costs, the incremental ones, now and in the future, when you consider a project. Ignore sunk and committed costs and think about opportunity cost as well. We ignored inflation for the sake of a simple example, but you should not if you're considering a project that extends over many years.

Chapter 8: Accounting

A big yawn usually accompanies a discussion of accounting. But the language of accounting is the language of business. After several years of practice, I joined the board of our veterinary association. At each meeting, they kept passing around these statements with numbers on them, income statements and balance sheets that showed credits and debits and the like. I had very little understanding of these issues then. Only after much study and time did I have an appreciation for the importance of these reports.

Two types of accounting are done. The first is financial accounting, aimed at the world outside a business entity and consisting of the reports that communicate to analysts and others the financial status of a business. The other is managerial accounting, discussed in the next section. It has an internal focus and allows those on the inside of a business to plan, control, and achieve the goals of the organization.

Financial Accounting

There are four types of financial statements, but we will discuss only two: the balance sheet and the income statement. These are the most commonly presented at meetings and the most relevant.

Balance Sheet

The balance sheet gives the status of an entity at a given point in time, usually once a year. If you look at the annual reports of the companies in which you own stock, you will see a balance sheet early on in the report. If you are on the board of a nonprofit or a for-profit business, you will see one of these at least once a year. In its most simple form, you will see the following:

BALANCE SHEET	
ASSETS	LIABILITIES
Current Assets	Current Liabilities
Long-Term Assets	Long-Term Liabilities
	Equity

Assets are just what you think: the items of value owned by the entity. The liabilities are the claims against those assets. Equities represent the claims of the owners, the shareholders. A simple equation governs these. Assets equals the sum of the liabilities and equity. Moreover, for a viable organization, assets must be of greater value than liabilities.

In a veterinary practice, current assets would consist of, at a minimum, accounts receivable and cash in the bank while long-term assets would be any property the practice owns. Current liabilities would be bills you owe in the next month or so. Long-term liabilities would be the future payments on any mortgages or other long-term loans. A glance at the balance sheet for my practice showed that current assets consisted of deposits at banks, accounts receivable, and notes receivable in the short term. Fixed assets included the furniture, equipment, inventory, and depreciation. Current liabilities consisted of accounts payable and accrued payroll expenses, while the long-term liabilities were mainly notes payable over an extended period of time.

VETERINARY PRACTICE BALANCE SHEET—SIMPLE VERSION:	
ASSETS	LIABILITIES
Current Assets	**Current Liabilities**
Petty cash	Accounts payable
Accounts receivable	Notes payable—current portion
Inventory	Accrued payroll expense
Operating bank account	Accrued payroll tax expense
Long-term assets	**Long-term liabilities**
Medical equipment	Mortgage
Computer hardware	Notes payable
Furniture and fixtures	Equity

The more complex the organization, the more complicated and detailed the balance sheet, but the basic equation holds. Equities are depicted on the bottom right, in part to signify the order of repayment in the event of bankruptcy or financial trouble. In the case of a bankruptcy, the right side of the balance sheet is paid from top to bottom, starting at the top. So those holding short-term liabilities are paid before those holding long-term liabilities. The owners, the equity holders, get paid last, and in the case of most bankruptcies, are not paid at all.

In any given time period, current assets should be worth more than current liabilities. If you are on the board of an agency or company and liabilities outweigh assets in the current period, look out. Ask some questions.

Balance sheet accounting is much more complex than these short paragraphs would indicate. Weeks are spent on this in accounting courses. CPAs and attorneys spend a lot of time arguing about how a given topic should be presented. Next, we'll discuss a few of the factors involved.

Assets are listed at their acquisition value, the historical cost. If your practice bought a building twenty years ago, the purchase price is what goes on the balance sheet, even though the value of the building may be much greater at this point. A balance sheet presents financial transactions only. If a company makes a strategic acquisition that has not yet paid off, that value is not reflected. In the case of a veterinary practice, the most significant assets are the doctors and their income-generating potential, and there is no place on the balance sheet to list these. Many of the figures given are estimates, and all of them reflect the past, not the present or future. Finally, accounting rules allow alternative ways of calculating and presenting data.

Clearly, a quick glance at a balance sheet won't do it justice, and you won't be able to fully analyze one without extensive training. Yet you can take a superficial look with more understanding than previously and be able to ask a question or so as well.

Income Statement

Doctors can understand this one. It gives the net income, the bottom line, and should be part of any financial presentation. Sometimes a business can have lots of cash coming in but the income statement shows no net income or even a negative bottom line. How so? Depreciation is the answer. If a business pays taxes, how an asset is depreciated can make a huge difference. Depreciation is the yearly expense of a long-lived item such as a building or computer. If you buy a computer, accounting rules allow you to set aside (at least on paper) an amount equal to, for example, 20 percent of the purchase price so you can buy another one in five years. Depreciation goes on the income statement as an expense even though it didn't cost you those dollars during that period of time. This reduces or sometimes eliminates your net income and therefore your taxes. The rules are complex, and for some purchases the rules allow you to charge off a lot more in the first few years than later on. If you buy a building, you will receive a tax benefit from depreciation and your income tax bill will be reduced. Veterinary practices typically have little income tax anyway, and purchases or investments that can generate tax savings from depreciation should be done in partnerships or business entities outside the practice. In this way, a doctor's personal income tax can be lowered.

Managerial Accounting

Two topics in managerial accounting, cost accounting and performance evaluation, resonated with me after our group had wrestled with the issues for years.

Cost Accounting

In a veterinary group, the spectrum of cost accounting can range from none (put all the expenses in a pot and divide them equally) to the extreme of figuring how each expense item affects each doctor and charging accordingly. As you might imagine, dividing up the use of all the supplies that flow into the typical medical group's office daily, if done accurately, would be very expensive, and not worth the extra overhead. I have never heard of a group going to this extreme. Most groups use a formula they have derived over time, and a split that works for that particular group. The formula should be fair to the lower-income doctors but not penalize the higher-income doctors, and it should provide incentive to be productive as well as to cut costs. All should realize that the pain of doing without something, be it an expensive piece of disposable equipment or staff, will be rewarded when the take-home pay is higher. Just as important, a doctor should readily see that any extra effort in seeing more patients and adding to the top line will benefit that doctor as well as the group. You can be sure that a lot of debate has gone into whatever formula your group has adopted and that a lot of your meeting time over your practice lifetime will be devoted to this topic. If everyone in the group makes approximately the same income, splitting overhead dollars pro rata by the number of doctors makes sense. In a practice in which there is considerable variation in income, a straight percentage split is less fair, especially to the lower-income doctors. The higher-income producers like this arrangement because they pay the same amount as everyone else and it takes a much smaller percent of their gross income. On the other hand, allocating costs purely by income is unfair to the high producers since their gross dollars paid will be far higher than the low producers'.

Here is an example of how this might work: 35 percent of overhead is split pro rata by the number of doctors in the group. Thus if there are ten doctors, each would pay 10 percent of the 35 percent. The remaining 65 percent is split according to percentage of income. Thus, the doctor who brought in 20 percent of the income would pay 20 percent of the remaining 65 percent of costs. This mimics the real business world in which there are both fixed and variable expenses. It provides incentives to produce and grow your revenues, because you can achieve a lower overhead percentage by working harder. There is less direct incentive to cut costs, but everyone should be dedicated to this goal even in the absence of a dollar-for-dollar reduction in their own allocated costs.

Realize that there is no one correct method of cost allocation and any system produces debate and controversy. In the end, whatever works for your group and produces a minimum of contention is the best for your group, even if a business school professor may fault it from a theoretical perspective. Be careful about changing the formula. Most of these unique formulas, like the group's culture, have arisen over time and serve the group well. Changing things can lead to trouble.

Many times a given doctor will propose that the formula be tweaked, and he or she will have an ostensibly good reason. If you delve into the effects of such a tweak, magically enough, the proposing doctor will benefit financially by such a change and the change may hurt others in the group. Then you will know the real reason for that innocuous-sounding alteration of something that has served the group well. Likewise, a doctor may propose staff changes, usually to get rid of a position that doesn't serve that doctor but does help one of the others in the group. It's almost unprecedented for a doctor to propose a change that is harmful to his or her own take-home pay or level of staffing. There is always a real as well as a good reason for any of these ideas. Sometimes the idea is good and the group adopts it, but in my experience, most of these are seen as self-serving and the group rejects them.

Performance Evaluation

The second topic relevant to veterinary practice covered the area of internal reports, especially as they related to the ongoing evaluation of an employee's performance. First, another truism: what gets measured gets managed.

When your group's medical leadership meets with the managers, what do they look at? Overall profitability? Patient satisfaction? Employee turnover? Supply costs? Whatever you look at and have numbers to track will be handled over the next few weeks at the least. This leads to a repeat of a cliché—people do what you inspect, not what you expect. If you tell your manager you want to see lower supply costs but that manager knows you will never ask about that issue again, the manager will ignore it. You have to follow up on matters that are important and, when possible, tie compensation to meeting a given goal or several of them.

You should set challenging but achievable goals with a manager or other employee by sitting down and negotiating with them. You should make your expectations clear and measurable, periodically monitor the progress in meeting those markers, and keep to your word in tying compensation to them. If they make their numbers and are due a bonus, pay it. If they don't and come with a bunch of excuses and request a bonus anyway, don't pay it. (Apply this rule with reason, of course. If your periodic meetings have identified obstacles out of the control of your manager, you should have adjusted your expectations accordingly before the end of the reporting period.)

Performance evaluations should be tailored to the job description. Thus the evaluation for a technician should differ from that of the front-desk staff. You will not be doing all of these for everyone in a practice, but someone should. Consider spending fifteen minutes every quarter as opposed to an hour every year. Problems can be corrected sooner, and if they're not corrected, a problem employee can be fired with full and frequent documentation of the reasons for the dismissal. When the unemployment insurance investigator from the state comes to check, you will be glad for all the paperwork you have.

This is a difficult area, and I am covering only the highlights. You should be aware of what needs to be done, even if you're not doing it.

Chapter 9: Business Law

A course in business law doesn't make anyone a lawyer, so this discussion of the issues important to veterinary medicine won't make you one either. However, our review should make you aware of some important issues. Please bear in mind that this section should bring issues to light that will require legal advice when you tread in these areas. Good lawyers are worth their weight in gold.

Antitrust

How do you make sure the clients keep coming in your door? Go to your competitor and carve up the market. You handle the south side of town and she takes the north side. Keep out of the other's territory, and both of you can grow. You cultivate one set of clients and she gets another. You can do as you please with your territory.

How do you set fees? Get all the veterinarians in one room, figure out a price schedule, and agree that everyone uses the same schedule.

Somebody thought of these things years ago and lawmakers have already handled it. You can't carve up a market and you can't fix prices, at least with competitors. These actions violate the laws pertaining to antitrust, and they apply to veterinary practices as well. Courts have ruled that the practice of veterinary medicine has its business aspects. They want veterinarians to compete just like all businesses are supposed to.

Americans with Disabilities Act

You're six feet tall and building a new office space. You want all the countertops to be high enough that you don't have to lean over to look at a chart or write a note. You want a comfortable back at the end of the day. Just tell the architect, and it's done. It's your space, you're paying for it, so you should be able to have it just like you want it.

One of your employees, marginal at best, is losing her vision. Since she can't work effectively with you in seeing your charts or the computer, you can fire her so she can find a job where she can perform. Right? After all, you hired her to work in billing and collections, and if she can't do her job, you have the right to get someone who can.

As you might have guessed, this is wrong—at least on the first example and perhaps wrong on the second. A relatively recent law covers both questions. In 1990 Congress passed the Americans with Disabilities Act (ADA) and thereby put restrictions and regulations in place that determine many activities formerly unfettered. If you have more than fifteen employees, the act covers you. The Department of Justice website says, "The ADA prohibits discrimination in all employment practices, including job application procedures, hiring, firing, advancement, compensation, training, and other terms, conditions, and privileges of employment. It applies to recruitment, advertising, tenure, layoff, leave, fringe benefits, and all other employment-related activities."

The act applies to "qualified individuals with disabilities. . . . An individual with epilepsy, paralysis, HIV infection, AIDS, a substantial hearing or visual impairment, mental retardation, or a specific learning disability is covered." The details and explanations cover many pages and, by now, court decisions. The individual has to be able to perform the essential functions of the job, but you may have to make "reasonable" accommodations that allow this. If the person cannot perform the job, that's a different matter.

Architectural barriers to the disabled had to be accounted for in new construction. When building a new office, you have to take into account all of these changes. You cannot have all the counters be suitable for a person who is six feet tall. Why? In case one of the staff is wheelchair-bound. It turns out that not all counter space has to accommodate those with disabilities, only a certain specified percent.

If your employee develops a visual problem, you must make reasonable accommodations to allow that employee to perform the job, including providing another person to act as a reader. However, if the employee remains marginal and truly cannot perform, you can terminate employment. You can imagine what happens when the marginal employee believes himself to be a good employee and accuses you of firing him because he can't see.

The ADA covers what you can and cannot ask when you are interviewing potential hires, not only about them but their family as well. You cannot discriminate against someone who has a relative with a disability on the assumption that excessive leave will be required to care for that individual. You must post a notice about all this if you have more than fifteen employees.

Noncompetition Agreements

We have discussed these in some detail, giving the point of view of the group demanding that a young doctor sign a non-compete. We will add a few more details in this section. We take much of our guidance from the medical doctor world when it comes to these agreements. The *American Medical News* discussed this topic in 2005.[1] This article provides details of the Tennessee Supreme Court's invalidation of a clinic's non-compete contract with a departing doctor, ending twenty years of favorable treatment of such clauses in the state. The court felt that continued care for patients outweighed the business interest of the clinic. Yet these clauses continue in many jurisdictions. The AMA opposes them and deems unethical any agreement that is excessive in terms of geographic scope or duration.

There is wiggle room in most situations, and attorneys should review any agreement. One alternative is a non-solicitation agreement, outlining rules against contacting patients or hiring staff. Thus a veterinarian can set up practice in the same area, but will have to develop a patient base while observing the tenets of the agreement. This sounds good in theory but in practice is difficult to enforce, especially if the departing doctor holds a grudge. Therefore, many practices go with the more restrictive and easier to

---

1 Beth Wilson, "Tennessee Physician Wins Case on Non-Compete Clause," *American Medical News*, 22 Aug. 2005.

enforce noncompetition agreement that prohibits any type of practice within the prescribed area for a specified time.

The joining doctor should be clear on the obligations of these contracts and be prepared to honor them if the occasion arises. Court fights are expensive and extremely time-consuming; they are to be avoided at all costs by knowing what you're getting into and determining ahead of time that you can live with the consequences of whatever you sign. In most litigation between doctors, no matter which side wins, both sides spend an inordinate amount of time and dollars to make a point, and the sure winners are the bank accounts of the attorneys.

Employment law is another area of great interest and also great disagreements between states. Consulting a lawyer to make sure you have all your documentation is essential. This is probably the area that most veterinarians get tripped up on. Most of us are nice people and want to help our staff, however sometimes the staff will take advantage of your kindness. There are countless stories of employees being caught for stealing from veterinary practices where the owners allowed them to stay employed. Most of the employers felt sorry for the individuals and wanted to help them. As payback for their kindness, the employees sued them for everything from discrimination, hostile work environment, to sexual assault. So consult your lawyer and deal with any employee issues straight on.

There are also many other smaller legal issues that we deal with every day, and each state is different. One example is keeping someone's pet if they do not pay their bill. Some states allow this, but many times you not only end up with a pet to care for, but an unpaid bill. Other issues I deal with frequently are bad checks, abandoned pets, and stray animals. As you can see, having good legal counsel is very important.

Summary

We have just touched on a few of the aspects of business law that affect the daily life of veterinarians, not to give legal advice in any way, but to alert you to issues about which you need to know and consult with attorneys. Most attorneys, like most doctors, are competent, well-meaning, and helpful. You should consult an attorney earlier rather than later. If you're writing a sensitive letter about a potential legal situation, clear it with your lawyer before you send it. If you're faced with a contract, talk to your attorney before you sign it, not after. As smart as you are, you don't have legal training, and seemingly innocent clauses in a letter or contract can come to haunt you if you unwittingly commit yourself to something you later regret.

Attorneys are very specialized, at least in the big firms. You should be sure to deal with a lawyer with veterinary experience in most of your affairs, yet when it comes to a will or setting up a trust, get a specialist. Litigators are a special breed, the pit bulls of the attorney world, and you want a mean one on your side. When we say "mean," we mean aggressive, tough, and willing to argue every point. If you have determined that you are going to war (litigation) on an issue, don't do it unless you mean to win and are willing to spend some money. If so, your hiring of a litigator signals your intentions. Most of all it is best to avoid litigation if at all possible.

Chapter 10: Operations Management

Efficiency is a very important part of business, and many veterinary practices are not great at efficiency. Why? The veterinarians in charge feel they can do a job better than the staff. Let's take a minute to look at a couple areas of efficiency.

Worry Curve

You have a project due, perhaps a paper you and a faculty member are writing together, where you're doing most of the work. The research completed, you agree that you will produce a first draft in six months. You can proceed in one of two ways.

First Scenario

Throw the research papers in a file and plan to get ideas on background literature to review in a few weeks. Every few weeks, look at the file and plan to ask about those papers to review. Then you will write an outline for your paper, let it stew for a while, and start to write. You worry a little bit. Proceed on this cycle for several months—after all, you have six months, and you're busy getting going with your new practice. As the first four months end, look again at that pile and begin to worry more. After five months, you worry a lot and get down to work, putting in late hours of reading and writing. At the six-month mark, you get an extension from your colleague, and after eight months, you finish the draft.

Second Scenario

Sit down with your faculty member and get some reading material. Get your calendar out and plan the project week by week. You worry a good bit about how to make it happen, so you think and think, write out your schedule realistically, and each week complete the tasks. At three months, you're halfway through and you're worrying less. At five months, you're almost done and the worry factor has gone away. At six months, you produce the draft on time.

Clearly, the second scenario is the way to go. Attack a project with planning early on. Do the worrying early and write a schedule you can keep, and then keep it. Overall, you worry less and you're more productive.

Efficiency

You like to spend time with your patients—after all, that's why you went into veterinary medicine. So you make sure you cover all the bases with each patient, chat with each client, and write out all the prescriptions and go over the instructions. In the first few months of your practice, this works great. Then you get a few more patients on your schedule and you start to get behind by mid-morning. You never catch up, and you're hearing complaints all afternoon, from clients and staff. You wonder why, since you're delivering far more personal care than others, those old guys who see more patients and move their days along. The clients' complaints get worse, and you get more frustrated.

What's going on? You're inefficient, that's what. After awhile, it begins to hurt. Remember that clients want time, but not necessarily all of it with you. They lump all the time they spend in the office encounter and consider this as time spent with you. So if you have an assistant write the prescriptions and go over the written instructions—printed instructions, not handwritten—you get the credit, and you could be in the room with someone else. You can see more patients (within reason), get each one out on time, and get better client satisfaction if you're efficient.

Efficiency begins when the client first makes an appointment. Before the appointment, do they get forms to fill out and a map to your office, or, better still, can they do this online? Are they told what time to arrive and how long to expect the visit to be? When they arrive, is there a long line? Do you have staff do all the things staff can do: move patients, routine instructions, diagnostic testing, etc.? How about checkout? Do you collect money for the bills quickly?

These are just a few of the issues concerned with efficiency. If you joined a group, perhaps they have already spent time on these items, but not necessarily. It took our practice years and concerted effort by the veterinary leadership and top staff to reduce lines at our check-in stations and to figure out the best way for our clients to exit. Efficiency demands attention and effort—not just once, but all the time. You can make all the rules and processes you want, but if someone doesn't make sure they're followed, in time they will be ignored.

Chapter 11: Corporate Finance

Two topics in this course resonated with us: the time value of money and investing.

Time Value of Money

Remember the instructions we gave about pension planning from day one? The magic of compounding? These relate to the time value of money. Which would you rather have: $1,000 today or three years from now? Which is worth more, and how much? If you win the lottery for $1 million and want to collect today, will you get a million dollars?

You know, or should know intuitively, that a dollar today is worth more than a dollar a year from now. Inflation and time erode the value of money so that any amount in hand today is worth more than in the future. The value of a sum today as compared to its value in the future depends on the discount rate, an interest rate made as an assumption. The factors going in to that assumption depend on current interest rates and the riskiness of the venture. Time matters also, as no matter the rate, the further into the future, the less a given amount today will be worth. Discounting is the process of computing the present value of a future sum of money, and the discount rate plays the key role. For example, at a discount rate of 6 percent, $500 five years from now is worth $373 today, while the same $500 is worth only $249 at a discount rate of 15 percent.

So how does this work in real life? That lottery payout of a million dollars is not the promise of a million dollars right after you claim the prize, but the promised payment is, for example, $100,000 a year for ten years. That's a million dollars, correct? Correct, if you ignore the time value of money. If you go to the lottery office and ask for a lump sum payment, you will get a lot less, because the lottery office will take each year's payment of $100,000 and discount the payment for each year back to today at a rate they choose. At a rate of 8 percent, $100,000 payable in one year is worth $92,593 today, and a payment scheduled for five years from now is currently worth $68,058. Calculating the value of each future payment back to today's value gives you the NPV: the net present value. Look at the table. You will see that the discount rate matters a lot. The higher the rate, the less a future payment is worth today. Setting the

The value of $100,000, promised in each of the next five years, when paid today. Two different interest rates:

NPV	8%	4%
Year one	$92,593	$96,154
Year two	$85,734	$92,456
Year three	$79,383	$88,900
Year four	$73,503	$85,480
Year five	$68,058	$82,193

discount rate can be contentious, but it should bear some resemblance to current interest rates and the cost of capital.

So how does this apply to veterinary medicine? As you build your net worth and your financial enterprise, you will attract a number of people—friends and supposed friends—who will want you to invest various things. Be aware of what happens to the value of money. Ask what the net present value of the investment is and what discount rate they used. After the jaws drop and they recover from the fright of a doctor asking a relevant business question, they may stammer a bit and equivocate. They will certainly respect you more and learn they can't put anything past you. You will learn more of the true value of the proposed investment.

Here's another example to illustrate the importance of interest rates. You, like most veterinary students, have debt from your school days and now you have to pay it back. Assume you owe $100,000, the interest rate at the time you borrowed the money was 6 percent, and you must begin monthly payments. Your monthly payments are $1,933 and the total you will pay is $115,980. But you're in a practice now and you have a private banker who's willing to let you refinance your loan at a lower interest rate, say 4 percent. Now your monthly payment is $1,842 and the new total is $110,520. You will save more than $5,000 by getting a lower rate. You can type "loan calculator" or "net present value calculator" into an Internet search and you will see a number of ways to play with these numbers.

Let's say that you know you must begin paying back that $100,000 five years from now, but your spouse is working and you're generating some extra cash each year. You want to save now so it won't be a strain in five years. The financially naive person might think, *Let's just save $20,000 a year and be done with it.* But you ask what a reasonable discount rate is and determine the net present value of paying $20,000 five years from now. At 6 percent, $20,000 five years from now is valued now at $14, 945, and at a 4 percent discount rate the present value is $16,438. So, assuming you can get these rates with a conservative investment, you only need to put aside the net present value of the future payment.

The flip side of discounting is compounding. Compounding gives you the future value of a sum of money today. Here again, the rate you choose determines the future value, and obviously, the higher the rate, the greater the future value. Just as important is time. The longer the time period, the greater the future value, and the last few years produce so much more value that it seems exponential. Hence our advice to begin pension saving as soon as you begin practice. You want compounding to begin working for you in your thirties.

You can find tables that allow you to plug in a rate and the number of years so that you can calculate these values exactly. Here's a rough rule that allows a quick calculation. Divide a rate into seventy-two and you will get the years to doubling. An investment that appreciates at 6 percent annually will double in roughly twelve years (seventy-two divided by six). An inflation rate of 4 percent will halve the value of today's dollar in about eighteen years (seventy-two divided by four). If you save $10,000 this year and it appreciates at 6 percent, it will be worth $20,000 in twelve years, $40,000 in twenty-four years, and $80,000 in thirty-six years by this rough rule. But you can't ignore inflation, the factor that gnaws away at the value of the dollar, so you will have to consult a table that takes assumed inflation into account. If the mythical average person retires at age sixty-five with a certain nest egg and lives another eighteen years, inflation can rob them of a further one-third to one-half of that nest egg. It's better to have a big nest egg if you're that average person.

Investing

You're smart, and now you have time to read the business pages. You're taking our advice about saving and you plan to invest your money yourself and do a lot better than the average guy. You've done some reading and you know that stocks provide the best returns over time, so that's how you're going to make a killing. What are your chances? Can you beat the market? Can you do better than your neighbor the stockbroker who spends all day doing this and has the added advantage of research done by his company? Can you know more than the hundreds of stock analysts around the country who constantly scour all sources of information about the companies they cover? It's possible. This does happen to the rare and very astute doctor, but be honest, is that you? In general, the odds are very much against you, and if you're truly smart, you'll realize your limitations and get professional help. The stock market and real estate crash of 2008 show that even professionals can't predict the downturns.

One of your friends, or even a relative, comes to you with an investing opportunity. It sounds great, it can't lose, and all you have to do is put some money in, sit back and, in a few years, rake in the dollars. A few questions: Why you? If this is such a great deal, why aren't the big guys offered it, and why haven't they already put their money in? How much is your sponsor putting in, and will he get a fee if you invest? When can you get out if you decide you want to? What's the track record of the person heading up the venture? Does it sound too good to be true? If a friend or relative is the sponsor, what if things go sour? Will lost money and hard feelings jeopardize a relationship? Consider the downside in all its dimensions, not just lost dollars, before going down such a path.

Some of these small privately offered, local ventures work. Most don't. If something sounds too good to be true, it usually is. Be careful. If you're reading this book, perhaps you already know your limitations and, if so, good. You should have a conservative accountant whom you trust, as well as an attorney. Run any proposed private ventures by them and follow their advice. If you're hell-bent on a particular investment, make sure you can afford to lose the dollars and make sure your initial investment is all you owe. I repeat: make sure your initial investment is all you owe. Do not commit to any more than your initial investment. Do not allow your name to be used as an officer or director of this venture without the full approval of your attorney, accountant, banker, and spouse. If taxes aren't paid or other problems occur, guess who they come after: officers and directors. Take notes, keep all documents for a long time, and be sure you understand the tax implications of any of these transactions.

These are real-life problems once you start accumulating net worth. You will have to decide how to invest your savings unless you practice in a big group that can afford to buy advice for everyone. Even then, you may have the option to carve out your dollars, and if so, you will be tempted as time goes by to see if you can do better than your advisor. When you're in a favorable business cycle, you will hear friends bragging about how much they made in a particular stock and you will see others strike it rich in real estate and other ventures. Remember that business cycles are just that, not a relentless slope upward. When the downturn comes, you may appreciate the steady, even income most veterinarians enjoy, and you will see some highfliers go broke.

Consistent, winning investment strategies are difficult. If you're business-minded, willing to study and take risks, and willing to take the blame when you lose, then perhaps personal investing is for you. For most veterinarians, investing should be left to professionals. Even then, you will have to provide direction and oversight. You will need to be aware of the issues involved in investing and have a strategy—you just won't be making the tactical decisions about which stock to buy, etc. The events of 2008, in which the stock market lost value sharply, credit contracted, and many people lost large parts of their net worth, demonstrate even more the importance of personal oversight of investment advisors. Keep written records, especially of instructions to your advisors, monitor results, and ask questions. You simply cannot be passive and blindly trusting.

Investing Strategy
Many good books address this subject, and what follows are general principles to consider.

Be Conservative

The dollars left after paying overhead, taxes, and essentials are precious. They go for fun and investing. If you don't have enough left over, look at what you consider to be essential. Fine wine, expensive vacations, and lots of dinners out are not essential. These should come only after you have put aside pre- and post-tax dollars for your future needs. Being conservative means not going for the high-risk investments, even if those have high rewards, which they sometimes do. When you're young and have many years for compounding to work for you, a reasonable return is all you need. So most of what gets invested for you should aim to provide this reasonable return in an investment vehicle that has a low chance of being lost. That said, you are in a better position to lose than people in their late fifties, so you can invest a small percent of your portfolio in higher-risk investments. This speaks to the next principle: diversity.

Diversity

You know the cliché: don't put all your eggs in one basket. This is good advice for you or your advisor. Stocks do provide the best return, but you shouldn't have all your money in stocks, and your dollars devoted to stocks should cover the spectrum of large cap, small cap, growth, value, domestic, international, and so on. As you get older, the risk profile should slowly swing more and more to safe investments, bonds, etc. Every book has a formula for all this. You need to know the principles and make sure your advisor follows a reasonable set of rules.

So can you do better than the pros? Should you pay for such professional advice or just get into an index fund?

Here's an unfortunate truth about professional advice: the best advice is expensive and unavailable to you early in your investing career. When your dollars to invest are small, i.e., in the tens or even hundreds of thousands of dollars, you simply can't get the same advice the big funds get. You will get the stockbroker who will rely on the advice and research of his or her firm. Some of these may be excellent and skilled enough to rival the results of the big funds. Many will not be. How can you know? If you were reading the business pages in the 1990s, you would have read of the unconscionable conflicts of interest that swayed the "research" of firms with the best reputations. You would have seen the investment banks' internal e-mails mocking the idiots who followed the official advice they promulgated. You would have read that those calls from the stockbroker with hot tips and great buys were like the specials pushed on you by zealous waiters: they represented what management wanted to sell at any particular time, not necessarily a great investment. You would have been turned off by the whole process.

Until you have a net worth in the millions of dollars, you will not be able to hear the advice of the very top people in the investing world. If you have a big group with a large amount of dollars to be invested, you may be able to get close to the advice and management given to those with tens of millions of dollars. Does that mean you will get bad advice? Probably not, but you won't get the best either, and you need to know it. You need to manage the process and make sure your advisor knows of your desire for a conservative, low-risk portfolio. After you meet, make notes and put in writing what you have agreed on and send it to the advisor.

If you're one of the unfortunate few for whom money is lost and you want to sue, you will need written proof of your instructions. You probably won't be picking the individual stocks—at least if you've carefully read the preceding paragraphs, but you need to monitor the results. The report sent to you each month or quarter should include a benchmark index. Is your portfolio outpacing the benchmark, even after fees? You can't necessarily expect this each month or quarter, but if you're not exceeding the appropriate index over time, change advisors or investment firms.

Don't be nice. Don't be rude, but don't sit back and suffer poor returns because you like the advisor or you get taken to play golf or to the professional baseball game. This is your retirement and your lifeline in case of disability. You worked hard to make these dollars and you're sacrificing current fun to save the dollars. Make sure they're working for you, and insist on getting a reasonable return.

What if your advisor is a good friend or family member? Now you may have a problem. Before you hire a close friend or family member—and you may well be tempted to do so on a number of occasions—consider what you will do if you're unhappy with the outcome. Can or will you fire this person? You will be extremely lucky if people you hire for anything—money management, home decoration, home-building project, lawn service, whatever—make you happy and satisfied with their performance over time. When you see a project or job done poorly, can you yell at the person or people responsible and make them correct defects or go away? You can if that's the only relationship you have with them; you may not be able to if it's your sister-in-law or cousin. Be very careful before you hire a relative or friend. The odds are you will either strain the relationship or have to put up with a suboptimal result. It may be better to make a policy that you never hire people close to you.

While you want a conservative portfolio, the risk profile should change over time. Early on, when you have the ability to overcome losses, your profile should be relatively riskier, which usually means more stocks than bonds and some amount of riskier stocks. Some advisors argue that the profile should stay like this even in your retirement, but the majority of advisors say to increase the bond percentage as you get into your late fifties and sixties. What about the really risky investments, the kind you will be offered by your acquaintances and friends? As long as you understand the risk, can lose the money, and make these a very small part of your overall portfolio, we see no problem. Make sure you can get a tax deduction for your losses, so don't use pension or 401(k) dollars. Remember that your pension dollars offer you such great opportunity because they are not taxed. This is the best tax shelter you will have, at least with current tax laws.

I hesitate to give investment advice, but the lessons I take away from my experience and education, in addition to the aforementioned, are to put all the dollars you can into tax-deferred vehicles, then:

1. Diversify into multiple investment buckets
2. Vary the risk profile according to age
3. Hire the best manager you can
4. Pay the lowest fees you can

5. Monitor and switch when necessary. Inspect what you expect, i.e., read those reports and make sure your manager(s) know you're keeping a watch.
6. If nobody can beat the indices, quit paying fees and invest in the index fund for each bucket.

Real Estate

What about real estate? We assume that you own your home or soon will, since that is a great investment in terms of personal life and growth in net worth. Buying other types of property can be fun and can make money; moreover, some investments have tax-sheltering features as well. If you go down this path, be sure it's fun for you. If you like the countryside, buying rural property or a farm can afford you enjoyment and growth in net worth. If you like prowling neighborhoods for good buys and, again, have the time to manage properties, residential real estate can make money for you. Here again, numerous books and seminars devote themselves to this area, and you would need to do your research and be committed. The drastic loss of value in the real estate world that began in 2008 demonstrates that such investments don't always hold their value. Real estate is cyclical, and so are other forms of business. Restrain yourself in the good times and don't be afraid to invest in the down times.

Do you own or rent your office? I rented our first office for seven years but invested in real estate and owned the building and the land when we moved. It's just like owning your home instead of renting: you're paying rent to yourself while the underlying property goes up in value. Assuming you feel good about the stability of your practice, owning your office space makes a lot of sense.

Chapter 12: Ethics

The rules of ethics concern treatment of patients, clients, competence of doctors, fees charged, and identification of deficient doctors. A doctor should place the welfare of the patient above all other considerations. The consideration of a patient's well-being should be paramount in all that we do, but sometimes, unlike human doctors, you have to factor in other concerns of the client.

Most veterinarians are ethical people. They did not choose this field because of the short hours and high wages. They chose this profession because of their dedication to helping animals and also people. However, sometimes running a business and the financial pressure of running a business can cloud people's medical judgment, leading to the running of extra tests, the prescription of extra medications, or even, in the worst cases, to the performance of unnecessary surgery. However, remember that financial success always follows good medicine.

The other interesting area of ethics in our profession lies in balancing the needs of the patients with the needs or constraints of their owners. There are many instances where the pet may need a surgery and the owners may not be able to afford or be able to perform the aftercare needed to make it a successful surgery. How do you handle those situations? Take, for example, a young, energetic two-year-old lab that ruptures his cruciate ligament. The owner has twins younger than two and is expecting her third child. Her husband travels all week, and she is the only one at home. Can she do the aftercare needed to make the cruciate repair a successful surgery? Some veterinarians will say, "That is not my problem. My concern is only to get the dog fixed." This is where we get into some moral dilemmas. Do we still suggest the surgery and let her worry about the aftercare? Do we postpone the surgery until we can better deal with the aftercare? What do we do to help this animal and this client?

How do you handle situations where owners are not seeing the reality of their pet's disease and are keeping the pet suffering unnecessarily? How do you talk to clients about this situation?

How do you handle times where you inform clients of the potential risks of a surgery only to have them threaten to sue you when their pet does not make it through surgery? How do you handle it when they refuse to pay because the pet did not live? How do you collect the money for all the service you rendered in these situations?

How do you deal with abusive clients? How do you deal with clients who say derogatory things to your staff? Do you dismiss a client, knowing that his or her pet will most likely not get any medical care if you ask this client to leave your practice?

All of these are very difficult ethical issues we deal with on a daily basis. There is not one answer to these questions, and the best path is to look at every situation and have an open discussion with the client and document the discussion. At some point you will probably have to make the decision whether you are in this profession to help just the animal, and the people are on their own, or if you are in this profession also to help people solve their animal problems. Both of these philosophies of our profession are correct, but depending where you fall, it will alter your decisions and discussion with the owners. I personally tend to fall into the idea that we are in the people business to solve their animal problems. I try to look at the whole situation and work with the owners to figure out the best plan for their animal. The only time that different philosophies might be a problem is when they occur in the same practice. If a client sees one doctor who is only concerned about the pet and then sees me, who tends to look at the whole picture, they might receive differing opinions on how to proceed with treatment. When owners receive conflicting treatment options, they get confused. Most clients think that there is only one way to treat medical problems, and if there are different opinions, they naturally tend to think one doctor is wrong and incompetent.

Ethics in our profession are difficult and ever-changing. We have to deal with the issues of pets as well as owners. Having veterinary friends and confidants can be invaluable when dealing with these issues.

PART III: YOUR CAREER

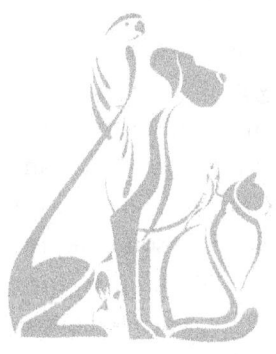

Chapter 13: Issues in the Early Years

Strategic Thinking

Think of this subject as the worry curve of your life, personal and professional. If you have followed our advice, you have already done some strategic thinking, perhaps without calling it such, as you contemplated where you wanted to be ten years from starting practice. The more you plan ahead, anticipating where you want to be and making the moves to get you there, the more you're doing strategic planning. Plan now. Settle some big issues at this stage of your career. Doing so will keep you from a lot of worries even later in your career, when you have even more at stake than you do now and solving problems is much more difficult. So consider the following questions now and address any problems that may be revealed. Did you make the following decisions correctly for you and your family?

1. Going into veterinary medicine in the first place: did you do this for yourself or your parents? Do you like veterinary medicine? Do you want to do this for the rest of your life?
2. Going into your particular specialty: did you choose your specialty for yourself or someone else? Do you enjoy treating this set of diseases? Seeing this type of patient?

3. Did you choose the right mode of practice—private vs. corporate vs. academic?
4. How safe is your specialty—will technology make your services moot or less needed?
5. Did you choose the right place to live? Would you or your family be happier somewhere else?
6. If your spouse has a career, ask the same set of questions. Both of you will need to be comfortable after your early years in the real world.

If the answers to these questions reveal that you are on the wrong path, the earlier you correct your path, the happier and more productive you will be. Many veterinarians find their way into law, the consulting industry, especially pharmaceutical and device companies, public health, and other careers. You may be committed to your present course for a year or so, but the sooner you plan your escape, the better.

Financial Planning

We covered this topic in detail in chapter three. Look back over those pages. Have you done what you should have? Consolidated student debt? Are you contributing to your retirement plan, fully insured, and saving some after-tax dollars? Perhaps you simply didn't have enough income to do all that you should have done back when you were getting started. If so, hopefully you now do, assuming you haven't let your spending habits get out of control. Remember the lessons of compounding and begin the proper financial planning now if you neglected it earlier.

Chapter 14: Are You Headed in the Right Direction?

Check Your Strategic Plan

You made long-term plans years ago—develop the career of your choice, grow a happy family, build up a good net worth, plan for retirement, and others. Where do you stand? Is this what you wanted, now that you have it? Are you and your family happy? Do you have a good balance between work, family, and recreational activity? Now is the time to revisit these issues. Even if you're in your late forties or early fifties, you can change things if it turns out you don't like what you have built for yourself.

Financial Planning

Have you saved? You can ramp up the effort for proper financial planning if you haven't done what you should have years ago. It's not too late, but you need to honestly assess your situation and commit to make changes if necessary. You don't want to wake up in your mid-sixties and regret your early and mid-career choices and actions. The financial press is full of stories about Americans not saving for retirement, and they quote an absurdly low level of money set aside by the average citizen. You're certainly not average, and your income is in the top 5 percent of US salaries, even if you may not make as much as you want.

But have you fallen into the trap we have warned against? You have to be brutally honest here. If you've fallen into the habit of spending all your disposable income and not saving, you know what you need to do. Cutting back your lifestyle in order to save for your later years is very hard. Pride and the fear of losing friends or status will keep most people in the trap they fell into. If you can't control your spending, you'll never recover. Earning a good income is the first step, and keeping some of it by not spending it all is just as hard as earning it. If you're in a hole, stop digging. Get help from a trusted advisor, whether it's from your accountant, banker, or a family member. Enforce a policy of saving, and make it happen.

Personal Planning

Are you content with your choice of practice type? If you're in academic veterinary medicine, where do you stand, personally and professionally? Does your work setting support your research and teaching efforts? Do you like your community? We hope the answer is affirmative on these and other questions you should be asking periodically. No situation is perfect, and negative features comprise part of any career choice. But do the positives outweigh the negatives? The same questions apply to your spouse and family.

What if the answers are negative? It's outside the scope of this book to deal with the various negative situations veterinarians may face, but here's the vision: you and your family should be in sync with each other, your work, and your community. You should be fulfilled by what you do and contributing to the welfare of those whom you serve. At the same time, you should be rewarded for your efforts and headed for the financial success appropriate to your choice of practice type and specialty.

If you, your spouse, or your children think you're unhappy, you should spend a good deal of time reflecting on and deciding the true cause of the unhappiness. You don't want to fix the wrong problem. If your discontent is personal and you blame your work setting and you change jobs, you will be just as unhappy. On the other hand, if you come home angry every day at your practice or your partner, you may need to move on, either to another community or to another practice setting. It's hard to admit you made a mistake all those years ago, but it happens, and it's not the end of the world. Now is the time to fix things.

Notice we used the phrase "think you're unhappy" above. Abraham Lincoln is reputed to have said that people are about as happy as they make their minds up to be. We long ago gave up on the idea of making our partners happy. We wanted a fair and equitable practice situation with decisions made for the welfare of the practice; happiness was a personal problem. So if you come home angry every day and you think it's your partners or your practice situation, somehow you need to be sure that you're not the problem before you make any disruptive changes. I see a lot of unhappy veterinarians and, without being their psychiatrist, I am reasonably sure that personal, not external, factors cause their discontent. Counseling may be the answer here, not a job change.

If you're sure that external factors are the problem, be sure you identify exactly what those factors are and then assess the impact of a change. If you made the wrong decision about the type of practice you want, what's involved with a change? Can you afford the income hit of a change? If the community is the problem, will moving solve things? Will you be able to replicate your work situation in a new place? Will any change truly improve things or just substitute one set of problems for another set, equal to those you're trying to escape? Be diligent and spend a lot of time planning, then make your move.

Burnout

You've been practicing or doing academics for years now, and there's a lot of routine stuff to face. Things aren't as new or challenging now that you have been doing them for so long. Yet you're busy, and your desire to succeed financially makes you over schedule yourself. You have a family that demands your time, and you manage the care for elderly parents. Everybody wants a piece of you, and all the days blur. You go, go, go but gradually lose the will to do so. Your motivation slowly ebbs, and it's a struggle to get going every day. You're always in a bad mood, and people begin to notice it. Hope has vanished, replaced by a long plateau of dreary days. A little of this is natural; a lot of this is a problem, and frequently burnout is the correct diagnosis, not necessarily depression.

As with all problems in veterinary medicine, you must make the proper diagnosis before you can start treatment, and you may well need help if some of the aforementioned problems are happening to you. Your spouse certainly can (and undoubtedly will) point out the problems in your behavior, but you may need professional help in sorting out exactly what's going on. If you're depressed, you will need help for this specific problem, and possibly medication. If you're burning out, a likely problem for veterinarians, you will need to reclaim your life in some way. Shed some responsibilities, schedule time off, exercise, meditate, or engage in other stress-reducing maneuvers. Unrelenting and excess stress leads to burnout, so you need to learn how to handle stress and use it for its good features. Managing stress properly will prolong your career and your life.

As you can see from this section, unhappiness stems from many causes: poor choice of practice, community, depression, burnout, and many others. If you're not satisfied, spend a lot of time (with help) deciding exactly what's going on before you make a corrective move.

Community Service

It may seem peculiar to follow a section on burnout with a discussion on something that eats up more of a doctor's precious time—community service—but we have a specific logic. Getting out in the community can serve as an antidote to a stress-filled, increasingly routine, and even dull practice. Serving on the board of a nonprofit agency, teaching, volunteering your services somewhere—any of these will help not only your city, but also you. We believe we owe something, and here's a way to give back.

In chapter three, we discussed why we should go out into the community. If you didn't do so early in your career, now may be the time.

What's in it for you? A break from routine and a chance to meet people you never would otherwise, perhaps gain new clients. It also gives you the opportunity to meet leaders of all kinds in your community, allowing you to establish connections in case you need some type of assistance in the future. Not to mention, it gives you the privilege of delving deeper into an area of interest while letting you learn how other organizations work or don't work.

What's in it for the profession? It gives you the opportunity to show the public another side of veterinary medicine—a personal side, a giving side.

Wealth Management

What can we, decided nonprofessionals in the areas of investing and money management, possibly say that hasn't been said by hundreds of books and magazine articles about managing wealth? Certainly nothing about the tactics of which stock or bond to buy, and not too much more than was already discussed in the section on investing in regard to strategy, or what buckets of investment vehicles to which you should allocate your dollars. But perhaps we can contribute to your vision of wealth and how you should think about your financial position.

Is your glass half empty or half full? If half empty, you look up the financial chain to the people making tens of millions of dollars with assets to match, and you feel pretty poor. If half full, you look the other way and feel pretty good. Veterinary medicine places us in at least the top 5 percent, if not the top 1 percent, of incomes nation- and worldwide. So yes, you're wealthy, or at least you're in the income range that should lead to wealth.

However, there are a few caveats. You need to pay attention to the lessons of this book. You need to work efficiently, utilizing whatever paraprofessionals are appropriate. So you may have to change your practice style over time. You need to watch your personal spending and contribute to your retirement. If you do all of these, you should leverage your well-above-average income into a considerable net worth and lots of choices as you go along. You will be wealthy by any standard. So what do you do in mid-career to keep things going?

Personal Maintenance

Take care of yourself! It's easy to ignore yourself when you're busy with a career, family, community, and other self-imposed duties. If you're in an academic setting, you have the added burden of research, teaching, and practicing enough to generate your income. And now, there's another time-consumer: you. You'll burn out if you don't take care of yourself, as we discussed in the section on burnout.

You're an asset. Yes, it may sound trite, but you are. Many people and entities have invested in you, even if you had to pay for some of your education costs personally. How much are you worth? You can figure your net worth, and you should periodically, especially because those pesky banks and other lenders will make you do so if you want a loan.

But how much are you worth as a conservative, money-generating asset to your family? Let's say your W-2 income is $175,000 and you wonder what amount of money in the bank would bring in that same amount. You should figure very conservatively, so assume you could get a consistent 5 percent return. You would need $3.5 million in financial assets to generate your salary. With inflation, you will need a little more each succeeding year. It's a very rare veterinarian who has generated that much liquid net worth. So you're an asset to yourself, who presumably likes the lifestyle your income affords, to your family, your partners or academic colleagues, and your community. They need you healthy and productive for many years, as do you. Many people depend on you to take care of yourself.

Are you overweight or are you fit? Look in the mirror and be honest. Is this your vision of yourself, or something that has snuck up on you as you've paid attention to other, seemingly more important things, like developing your career and juggling all the demands put on you?

Remember you are an asset to yourself and your family, and you need to take care of that asset.

Family

Part of a mid-career checkup should include an honest assessment of your family, including your relationship with your spouse and children. For most people, family assumes more and more importance, and to us, family is the most important. You're probably the primary breadwinner, but bringing in the bread, the bacon, and all that you can, is just the first of your duties. Do you spend time with your spouse, jointly planning the course of events? Do you spend time with your children? Do you read to them, or just let them play on the computer? When they're grown, will they look back on time spent with you or remember someone always working on their own thing? Spending time one-on-one with them will not only help them grow in the direction you want, but you will be repaid as you get older and you realize that *they are your most prized possessions.*

Vacation

Time off recharges you. Trips away from home bond families together and expand horizons. So travel within your means, but definitely go. Whether your trips are for long weekends or for weeks at a time, near home or outside of it, go. You won't regret it.

Hobbies

Does your career consume your life? Do you work all the time, squeeze in a few hours for family, and get back to it the next week? Does this happen week after week? If so, after years of this, the following thought insinuates itself into your brain mid-career: *Is this all there is to it? Work and nothing else?* This thought plagues just about everyone mid-career, veterinarian or not, but it will jump in with a vengeance if all you do is work. You have to find a balance. Family time and exercise are two ways to find balance, but a hobby or interest that's just for you is important as well. Your children will grow up and leave, you will retire someday, and you can't spend all the time with your spouse. Just as you should be preparing for retirement financially in ways already discussed, you should be preparing in other ways. When hard-charging people define their existence only by their profession and then retire, unhappiness, depression, or even premature death may happen. You don't want to be one of these. By the time you're in your forties, and especially when you get to your fifties, you've seen friends and family members die unexpectedly or, worse, develop disabling illnesses that force retirement at an early age.

For now, in mid-career, develop the vision for the rest of your life: increased financial security, and a balanced life with family time, hobbies, exercise, and community service. If you do these things, you'll be prepared for whatever comes, whether a long and productive career followed by retirement or a career cut short by illness and disability.

Chapter 15: Group Leadership

You've paid some dues in your practice, you've been there awhile, and all of a sudden, you're tapped for a leadership position. You're now the go-to person. People will come to you with all manners of questions and problems, big and small, and they will expect answers and solutions. How you handle these will communicate your leadership style and, over time, will determine the culture of your practice. Do your decisions reflect a desire to handle things expediently, with only the short term in mind, or do you follow a set of principles and let the long term rule? Does your practice have a strategic plan or blow with the wind, dealing with emergencies and urgencies? Do you force people to do things right, or just get the problem solved in whatever way works best?

Strategic Planning: Is Your Ship on the Right Course?

You are now in charge. Just as you have been developing a vision for yourself with the help of this book, you now need to check the vision for the practice. So you dust off the formal strategic plan that your practice determined a few years ago and start reading. But if the file is empty and no such plan exists, then your practice is in the majority.

Most do not have formal strategic plans that guide them year after year.

Should you have a plan and a vision, as well as ways to handle external and internal demands? You know the answer. Just as you need to know where you want to be in ten years in your personal life, so too does your group need the same thing.

If you're one of the few practices that have a plan, how old is it, and does it need to be updated? If you don't have one, make plans to develop one. When you're the leader and have to tell someone no to something, it's easier if you can refer to the will of the practice. Likewise, when you're in charge of prodding colleagues into action, it's easier if you can remind them that everyone agreed this was the way to go. We can attest to the value of this exercise, as can innumerable business leaders and thinkers.

Daily Administration: Keeping Your Ship on Course

Think of the following as our list of the activities that keep you going in the direction your practice decided it wanted to go. Most of the participants in that strategic planning process, unless they were given a specific job as part of the plan, will put that report in the drawer, forget it, and depend on you for execution. The fun part of strategic planning is the meeting where you do the thinking and you come up with the plan. The hard part is the basic blocking and tackling, making sure on a daily or weekly basis that you keep going. So keep your report on the desk where you can see it, and make things happen. It's your job now.

Efficient Operations

Do clients get checked in with all pertinent data captured in a timely way, so the folks in the back, waiting to see them, don't have to twiddle their thumbs? Do you use a website for registration and the making and changing of appointments? A walk through your reception area in the middle of any busy day will answer these questions.

Overhead

The practice will look to you when those yearly reports come out and overhead is recorded. Most of the time, attention is paid to the numerator of this equation, the expenses, and properly so. Controlling expenses takes weekly if not daily discipline. Most doctors want generous salaries and raises for the staff in their areas; after all, it makes life a lot easier. Likewise, these doctors are quick to advocate adding staff to make their days pass more easily. And, doctors being human, they are quick to point out perceived excess staff in areas outside their own and lobby for low raises for or elimination of these positions. Since staff expenses usually make up the largest part of any group's overhead, indulging in large raises and extra personnel is the path to overhead that's out of control.

You handle this by having a small group of doctors and senior staff—usually an executive committee if the practice is large enough—to monitor and approve staff raises and other aspects of expense control. You should know the community norms for each type of position, and your pay scales should match these norms, as should your yearly raises. It's hard to say no a lot, but you will have to if you want to keep expenses down. For your own peace, the committee should be handing out these nos, not you alone. If you are in practice alone, then you are the one to say no. However, if someone confronts you about a raise, always say, "Let me think about it." Agreeing to things right away will get you into trouble.

Overhead is a ratio of expenses divided by income, and some doctors conveniently forget that increased income will also lower that ratio. Does everybody pay attention to charges, making sure not to miss any? Do they give good estimates, let people know what the charges are, come up with different plans to help fit into the client's budget? Do the doctors work hard, seeing as many patients as they can while keeping them satisfied with great care?

Overhead reduction means paying attention to both the numerator (the expenses) as well as the denominator (the income). Each component of the ratio needs to be managed if a practice wants low overhead. If a doctor lags in production, you should have numbers that provide objective and authoritative data to help you make your case for decreasing his or her income. This is the same for expenses, staff, and otherwise. If a big push to lower expenses is necessary, you will get support from your colleagues more easily if you can convince them that a given area is out of the norm for a practice of your size and specialty.

Communications

If your practice is anything like mine, keeping everyone informed is a constant challenge, and this applies to staff as well as doctors. Good decisions are made, or poor decisions are properly overturned, but the team doesn't hear about it. Sometimes it's because they aren't paying attention, but frequently it's because you or your administrator omitted that last key step. You're busy—you're squeezing in administrative duties on top of seeing patients. You move on after making a decision, but you forget to let everyone know. It's human, but it bothers people, and it keeps your good work in making decisions from having the intended effect.

Every practice should try to have an administrator or executive whose job is to coordinate the staff and do some of this communication effort, but you will need to set up a system with that person to let not only the staff, but your fellow veterinarians, know what's going on. You will find that whether you use a formal newsletter, e-mail system, or electronic bulletin board, there will always be those who either never read it or skim and forget it. You won't escape the complaints about communications, but the best you can do is to set up a system that you can point to when the complaints come your way.

Continuing Established Policy

You may have made a great decision two years ago and the new policy may have been implemented for the first year or so. Then things slipped back to the way they were done before. Whether it's the way you collect information from patients or how you work in the exam room, inertia takes over and your policies gradually slip—unless you and your administrator keep a close watch and make sure things keep happening. It's not enough to set procedures; you have to follow up to be sure they're carried out at the beginning and periodically as time goes by. This is now part of your job, so be sure you tend to this as well.

Compliance

Depending on the legal structure of your group, you as president and CEO have specified legal duties and responsibilities. You should check with your lawyer. Even though many doctors, especially in small groups, consider the president of the group to be only the first among equals and not truly a leader, the law may have other things to say. You are responsible for compliance amongs many other duties and, for many reasons, need to keep a close watch in this area. Regulations, complex as they are, change. Your practice may be doing something in a manner that was correct two years ago but now is not. When you repeat one small (and innocent) mistake hundreds if not thousands of times, you can make a hungry investigator quite happy. Make sure you keep checking with the latest changes in the laws.

Running Meetings

We want to emphasize again the importance of ending a meeting on time. Nothing will make people appreciate your leadership more. They won't remember all your wise comments or great decisions, but if you get them out on time every time, they will remember you with great fondness. You owe it to them. It's not easy, but it can be done. You do it by being relentless on time: start on time, and keep to the subject on the agenda and the time allotted to it. (You did allot a time limit for each subject and wrote it on the agenda, didn't you?) You have to notice and call attention to it when the discussion gets circular and the same thing is being said for the third time. You have to cut off the long-winded ones and force a vote. In short, you have to lead the meeting. Your reward, in addition to more time in your own personal life, is gratitude. This is a commodity you will find in increasingly short supply as your leadership tenure continues.

Relationship with Your Colleagues

As the group's leader, you have significant organizational and legal responsibilities but, as you will find, nowhere near the authority and power as compared to CEOs in traditional corporations. Unless you're the leader of a huge practice, your board consists of fellow veterinarians who are independent-minded and over whom you have little direct control. You can't make them do anything, even things the group has voted as policy. You can't discipline them or punish them, and there will be times when you wish you could and the group suffers because you can't. Nevertheless, that's the reality.

So how do you deal with it? How do you deal with a veterinarian in your practice who is falling short in some area—patient care, documentation, or behavior? First, with the exception of a few pernicious types, just bringing attention to the behavior will influence most of your colleagues. If you call them on their actions, and especially if you have the practice's vote or policy on your side, they will comply. You have to do it, even though it's uncomfortable. You have to be direct but not obnoxious, and you can't use weasel words. Direct, clear communication will suffice with a good number of problems.

Problem Doctors

What do you do with problem doctors—those who seem to be causing trouble in some form or fashion and ignore your initial efforts to rectify things? First, act quickly. The other doctors in the practice will be quick to criticize such fellow doctors but slow to do anything more. They certainly won't take it on themselves to confront a problem, even if part of it is interpersonal. If you find out the facts quickly and point out the problem, if there is one, many times the situation is solved. The result of keeping quiet is continued damage to the reputation of the involved doctor, to the point that future problems are met with punishment that is out of proportion to the problem. Take action quickly and directly, and most doctors will correct their behavior. If they don't, you have learned something.

Get all the facts. There are always two sides to any story. No matter how convincing or damning one side of the story is, you should keep an open mind until you've heard the other side and have all the details. So tread carefully until you have all the facts and are aware of all the interpersonal biases and past history. Be aware that sociopaths take special pains to butter up those in power and then use their position of favor to undermine others in the group. If you're working with one of those, be careful if that doctor then starts to bash another colleague.

You should reread the section (see chapter five) about the various types of problem doctors a new practice member may face. If your practice is big enough, you as leader may confront some of these types and need to take action. Fortunately, they're rare, and most of your problems will deal with the squabbling of bright, driven, and independent-minded professionals, all of whom want their own way instantly.

If you think you have one of these significant problem doctors in your group, what should you do? First, take complaints seriously. Second, depending on circumstances and the size of your group, form a committee to look into the allegations. You will need the help and the support of this group if you have to propose action to your board or leadership group. Get as many details as you can from as many people as you can, and decide if you truly have a problem. Be fair to the accused doctor and don't assume the worst until you're sure. Have the support and advice of your attorney throughout this process.

Troublemakers and Abusers

Are you dealing with a personality problem or a troubled doctor who vents at the office because of hidden personal problems? Many of these people are basically good doctors going through a rough patch or who have depression or untreated adult attention deficit hyperactive disorder. If you have a chronically angry, passive-aggressive individual who can never change, do you get rid of that person or put up with him or her? Just as important, would your board support you, even if you decided someone had to go?

You're probably not a psychiatrist and not capable of making the crucial first-level cut of diagnosing whether you're dealing with a good doctor having personal problems or someone with a personality disorder. But this distinction is critical. After learning the extent of the disruptive behavior, a good first step is mandatory counseling of the doctor by a psychiatrist who, with the knowledge and consent of your doctor being treated, reports the findings and progress to you periodically. The disruptive behavior goes away, the doctor keeps his position, and the organization is happier and avoids the disruption of firing a professional. This approach is fair and gives a chance for the problem to resolve amicably. If the disruptive behavior continues, then you can take the next step—dismissal—with a clear conscience.

Incompetent Doctors

They exist, and come from all programs, even those with the best reputations in the world. The first step to dealing with this problem is prevention. As the leader, you will be in charge of recruiting new doctors to your group. Whether you're hiring a new doctor, nurse, assistant, or front desk staff, make sure to *do your homework*. Search firms call it due diligence, and it's vitally important. Check out the person, calling all the references provided by the candidate, and call other people—those not listed as references, if you know them—for candid assessments. You simply can't check with enough people. As time-consuming as it is, do it, and on occasion you will find out some things that will lead to your offering a job to someone besides your candidate. This will ultimately help you prevent future problems.

You have to listen carefully and read between the lines. Everyone is gun-shy of lawsuits, and they know that adverse comments may get them into trouble, so most people, unless you know them personally and they trust you, will not be forthcoming with a negative recommendation. You have to craft your question carefully and listen closely. What if you get the following response? "I'll be glad to tell you about this person, but I have a form they need to sign first, giving me clearance." Across the fax machine comes a detailed form for your candidate to sign, saying that they won't sue your informant no matter what is said, or legalese to that effect. You have your answer: your informant never said anything adverse, but the message is clear. It's saying that the person knows some negative things, so negative that the typical boilerplate permit for them to talk is not enough. So instead, they get your candidate to sign away all rights to sue, and then they can tell you whatever they want. It's a technique you can use if you fire a professional for incompetence and later get that phone call when he or she is looking for another job.

Well, say you did your homework and you hired a doctor, and a few months later, complaints from nurses, technicians, and other doctors in the group begin coming in. Sometimes it takes a year or longer, especially if it's after the probation period is over. As rare as it is, it happens. I have seen veterinarians from the absolute best programs, with great recommendations and compelling personalities, turn out to be marginally competent and not up to the standards of my practice. Sometimes you simply have to practice with someone for a significant period of time before you know. When you know, and you are sure, you have to act. As hard as it is, you have to let that person go. Be sure to have a contract worded in such a way that the group can do what's right. The leadership has to do the right thing for the protection of their patients and the reputation of the practice.

Here again, a fair process may be in order, depending on the circumstances. It may be that some advice from a senior doctor on a slightly different surgical technique or a different approach to certain patients can turn someone around, and I advocate trying this. If it's clear you have a lemon, don't waste your time, but in other cases, remediation can save a doctor from the shame of dismissal and, more important, lead to correct behavior in your group while avoiding bad behavior that otherwise would be perpetuated somewhere else.

Greedy Doctor

Most doctors want to do the right thing but may have gotten into bad billing or practice habits because of where they trained or previously practiced. As with the other types of troublesome situations, due process, a warning, and a chance to correct excessive actions will turn around a doctor who truly wants to do right. The indications for testing and surgery vary widely around the US, and someone whom you view as a "cowboy" may simply be practicing at the standards of his previous location or training. You find out by having a calm discussion with data and giving your firm expectation of a change in behavior. You will find out soon enough the type of person with whom you are concerned. The behavior will change in a good many instances, and your due process will have served the purpose of fairness and will have saved a basically good doctor, as well as your group, from the trauma of a forced exit.

If you have a truly greedy doctor on your hands, you will see that the excess billing, testing, or operating continues. Or that doctor may make plans to leave under circumstances of his or her own choosing, which usually means to the detriment of your group. That doctor may try to circumvent the non-compete you have in place by setting up a practice close to your office or by inducing key employees to leave. So be careful when you go down this path with any type of undesirable doctor. Get advice from your attorney, put everything in writing, and make sure to watch and move quickly if necessary. Do all of these as if you would be defending your actions in court, which you will be someday if your group is big enough and you do the right thing.

Lazy Doctor

Depending on the income split of your group, laziness can manifest itself in several ways, and the fix, if any, differs as well. If your group splits income based on individual productivity, some version of you-eat-what-you-kill, a lazy doctor just makes less. Magically enough, the drive to make more money cures this problem many times in such a situation. The exception would be the doctor who has income from a spouse or family and simply doesn't need the practice income to maintain lifestyle. In that case, you may be stuck with someone occupying a slot in your group in which a busier doctor would provide more care for patients and more contribution to overhead, leading to less stress on others in the group and a correspondingly lower overhead burden. What to do? This would be a group decision, based on how much you like the doctor, how much overhead sacrifice the rest of the group suffers, and how long the doctor has been in the group. There is no easy solution.

Sociopathic Doctor

As a group leader, you need to be aware of sociopaths. You should beware of super-charming people—those who talk a lot but don't say much. Sociopaths can be very intelligent and look on the surface like wonderful people. They butter up those in superior positions of power and spread poison about their peers. This serves them well when a peer catches on to them and reports them to the leadership, only to find that they are the suspects, not the sociopath. Leaders need to know human nature, the good and the bad. They need to be on their toes all the time and realize somewhere in the back of their minds that all is not what it seems to be sometimes. Take your time, get a group together, and investigate issues carefully before coming to a judgment.

Unless you're a psychiatrist, you may be on dangerous ground in making a diagnosis of a sociopath on your own, as the corollary of such a diagnosis is that you can't really trust anything that person says. Don't hesitate to get the professional help you need if you face such a situation.

Impaired Doctor

You cannot ignore this in a colleague. Here is another instance where at least one attempt at rehabilitation is correct. It may well turn a doctor around, and I have seen that happen, and it's only fair. On the other hand, you must protect patients and the group, and you should avail yourself of professional and legal advice.

Handling the Staff

While you may view yourself initially as your doctor colleagues do, a first among equals with little real power, your staff views you differently. You are the president and leader, the one they view as having a great amount of power.

They will pay more attention to you, and what you say to them will mean more than when you were "just" one of the doctors. Both praise and criticism now mean more, so you should be careful. Walk around more and observe. Let them all know you're looking and noticing. Set a good example in how you treat patients and others with respect and courtesy. Your behavior will begin to influence the group more than you know.

Keep your doors and your ears open. Don't assume your senior administrative staff is perfect, and listen to the issues from the front line. Show personal concern during times of illness and bereavement; write notes, make phone calls. You now represent your entire practice and can influence your staff's perceptions of all the doctors.

Miscellaneous Thoughts

As I briefly mentioned, don't assume that your job is to make your colleagues happy. George Orwell said, "Men can only be happy when they do not assume that the object of life is happiness." Abraham Lincoln is reputed to have said, "People are about as happy as they make their minds up to be." Veterinarians have many reasons to feel unhappy in the first decade of the twenty-first century: reduced fees, changing practice patterns, changing relationships with universities and referral hospitals, increased scrutiny and regulations, constant threat of lawsuits, and problem patients. We also have many reasons to feel happy: we are still respected in society, we help people with their animal problems, most of our clients like us, we earn a good income, we're solidly in the upper-middle class of society, and we're more independent than many professions. Happiness is up to the individual. Your job is to make your group fair, productive, and helpful to your patients and clients. If you fall into the trap of trying to make doctors happy, you will be very unhappy yourself.

Take time to make decisions. As Baltasar Gracián said, "Reconsider. Safety lies in looking things over twice . . . what was long desired is always more appreciated . . . let your 'no' ripen a bit . . . most of the time, the first heat of desire will have died down, and it will be easier to accept refusal."[1] This doesn't mean that you torture people and never make a decision, but think about things and get the other side of the story. When your answer is yes, you make the call. When your answer is no, let someone else deliver the bad news.

Late Career

You're in your sixties, you're healthy, your children are on their own, and you don't have to work as hard because you have a flush retirement plan as well as investments outside the plan that you can use to supplement your income. You have some choices finally, and you can do what you want within reason. Not all veterinarians will be this fortunate, but many will be, especially if they follow the guidelines outlined in this book.

---

1   Baltasar Gracián, *The Art of Worldly Wisdom*, Translated by Christopher Maurer, Bantam Doubleday, 1992: P. 74.

Chapter 16: Transition to Retirement

Transition and Slowing Down

If you do have these choices, now is when you can revisit the question that you presumably answered when you went into veterinary medicine: What do I want to do with the rest of my life? Did you really want to go into veterinary medicine in the first place? If you did then, do you still want to be in medicine? If you entered medicine for the wrong reason, do you want to escape? How do you really want to spend your time? If you know the answer and it's not practicing medicine, you may be able to make a change at this stage, when you have many years ahead of you. If you contemplated such a change earlier in your career, you may have found that the financial sacrifice of getting started in a totally new direction was too much for that stage of your life. Now it may not be. We can't tell you what to do, and many books purport to. You will need a lot of thinking and family consultation, if not professional counseling. At this stage of your life, you have fulfilled your obligations, and now it's your time. Do what you truly want to do.

On the other hand, you may realize that you like veterinary medicine and that you made the right decision in the first place, but you don't like the pace. If this is so, assuming your partners and practice type allow it, you can simply slow down. Work fewer hours in the day, see fewer patients in the same hours as before, or take more whole days off. Be sure you get a true picture of the financial consequences. Your income production will decrease, and depending on how office overhead is calculated, your personal overhead as a percentage of your income may increase, further depressing your take-home pay. Know what you're getting into. Be sure you can live with it, and then proceed as you wish. You've earned it.

Another consideration for some practice situations is the effect that slowing down will have on the value of your practice. If your ultimate exit plan is a sale of your practice, the diminished income resulting from a slower pace will reduce the price you can ask, since most practice valuations are calculated as a multiple of the income. Also consider that you may practice for more years in a slow-down mode than you would have if the only option were to work full time and then retire. Thus, the income generated by these extra years may offset or exceed the loss of value in your practice. Get some help in a full analysis of the impact of slowing down so you know you can live with the consequences, and do what you want.

Retirement

You're in your sixties and healthy, not thinking about retirement—you're too young, and many people work into their seventies these days. You've revisited your career choices, decided to stay in veterinary medicine, either at a full pace or somewhat reduced, and you're in the traces. Here's why you'll begin to at least think about retiring, even if you don't want to.

Your clients. Maybe you used to hear, "You look too young to be a doctor." Not anymore. Now you might hear, "You're not going to retire on me, are you?" or, "Tell me when you're going to retire so I can get my pet's surgery done before that time."

Your friends. They're starting to retire, voluntarily or involuntarily. Or they get sick or, worse, die. It's then that you might start thinking about all the things you've wanted to do and the places you wanted to see.

Your family. You have grandchildren, sometimes a distance away. You want to spend more time with them and other members of your family, hopefully even your spouse.

For all these and many other reasons, retirement will enter your thoughts more than you know. Does that mean you should retire? No. Slow down? Not unless you want to. But you will be thinking about it. In fact, if you've followed our advice, you've been preparing financially for retirement for years and you've branched out from medicine in your afterwork activities. You're better rounded than you were in training, and retirement is not a death sentence but a life choice. You will be thinking, but you don't have to act until you're ready. If your health or family considerations force you to retire earlier than you want, then you're ready, but hopefully the timing will be totally elective and all your choice.

However, your day of retiring will come. And when it does, we wish you the best and a long, healthy life after veterinary medicine when you enjoy your family, hobbies, and the fruits of your labor.

Other Books by Dr. Harbin

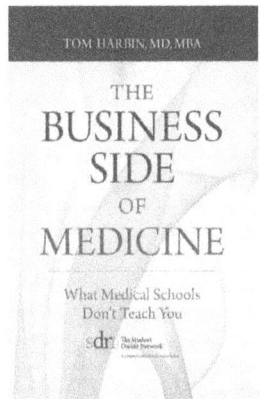

The Business Side of Medicine

Waking Up Blind - Lawsuits Over Eye Surgery

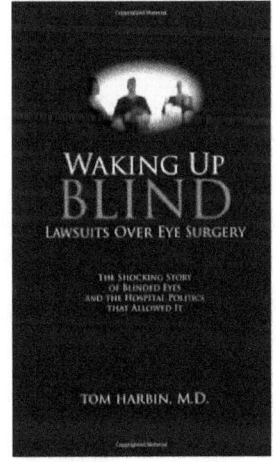

CPSIA information can be obtained
at www.ICGtesting.com
Printed in the USA
BVHW06s2055081018
529574BV00034B/3055/P